Praise for

THE VITALITY JOURNAL

"In *The Vitality Journal*, Dr. Deborah Zucker offers a compassionate invitation to come home to yourself—gently, at your own pace, and with deep respect for the wisdom of the body. This journal is a kindred resource for those healing from trauma, helping you to reconnect to your innate resilience, aliveness, and inner trust. *The Vitality Journal* is a gift on the journey to becoming whole."

—DR. ARIELLE SCHWARTZ,
clinical psychologist and author of *The Complex PTSD Workbook*

"In a time when self-care is perseverance, it's delightful to have a guide that helps us turn inward with joy!"

—AMY B. SCHER,
author of *How to Heal Yourself When No One Else Can*

"*The Vitality Journal* is a rare gem—both practically grounded and profoundly transformational. Dr. Deborah Zucker offers a living invitation into what I call 'whole-being healing,' where the sacred and the somatic are not split, but dance in intimate union. This journal doesn't just guide you back to your vitality, it welcomes you home to the radiant mystery of being fully, messily, beautifully human."

—SANIEL BONDER,
founder of Waking Down in Mutuality® and
author of *Healing the Spirit/Matter Split*

"Nearly 10 years ago, I had the privilege of writing the foreword for Dr. Deborah's book, *The Vitality Map*. Like that book, this journal offers direct and digestible suggestions for improving the condition of your life. In today's world of information overload, *The Vitality Journal* is a great way to start—clearing the old and resetting the mind for healing."

—MICHAEL B. FINKELSTEIN, MD, FACP, ABIHM,
author of *Slow Medicine*

"With wisdom, playfulness, and love, Dr. Deborah Zucker hosts a compelling exploration of what deeper health and freedom feel like from the inside. Each of the nine keys is like a long-forgotten room she helps us inhabit—awakening an interconnected weave of aliveness within. I plan to return to this journal again and again, to support lifelong inner adventuring, and true, multidimensional health."

—BROOKE MCNAMARA,
Zen teacher, poet, and author of *Feed Your Vow*

"In a world that often separates the spiritual from the physical, *The Vitality Journal* is a refreshing and necessary reminder that our bodies are not simply vessels—they are integral to any authentic journey of transformation. With depth, clarity, and compassion, Deborah invites readers into an integrative exploration that honors the dynamic interplay of body, mind, and spirit. I deeply appreciate how Deborah's approach addresses the whole person—supporting not only physical vitality but also creating the conditions for inner growth and wholeness."

—SARAH MARSHANK,
author and founder of Selfistry

"Knowledge without experience is valuable, but embodied learning—what I like to call wisdom—is even better! This book offers plenty of opportunities to transform knowledge into wisdom. Dr. Zucker's kind and compassionate voice shines through as she encourages readers to go at their own pace, practice what they've learned, and step into the next, greatest version of themselves with renewed vitality."

—DAVE MARKOWITZ,
author of *Self-Care for the Self-Aware*

"In *The Vitality Journal*, Dr. Deborah Zucker couriers you on a gentle, caring journey to uncover your authentic, meaningful life. Through journaling, inquiry, awareness, and playful curiosity, you shift from reactivity to conscious responding—and your inner guidance lights the way."

—JANETTI MAROTTA, PhD,
author of *50 Mindful Steps to Self-Esteem*

"In a world longing for transformation, *The Vitality Journal* offers the wisdom and action steps needed for true change. With keys like acknowledging our unique mortality, healing the shadow, and fostering resilience, Dr. Deborah guides us on an inner journey that ripples healing into our lives and the world. Join Dr. Deborah on this path of practical, actionable steps toward your best self and greatest life."

—KAREN M. WYATT, MD,
author of *7 Lessons for Living from the Dying*

"*The Vitality Journal* is an accessible guide to cultivating basic life skills to promote optimal health and wellness. By following the nine keys to deep vitality, readers can honor their uniqueness, strengthen their resilience, and improve self-awareness. At a time of global uncertainty, finding a path to health and healing is more important than ever."

—JAMES LAKE, MD,
author of *Integrative Mental Health Care*

THE
VITALITY
JOURNAL

9 KEYS TO
RECLAIM YOUR HEALTH,
INCREASE RESILIENCE,
AND CULTIVATE
JOYFUL SELF-CARE

The Official Companion to the Award-Winning
THE VITALITY MAP

DR. DEBORAH ZUCKER

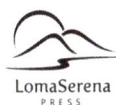

LomaSerena
PRESS

Contact
LomaSerena Press
info@lomaserenapress.com

Ordering Information
Special discounts are available on quantity purchases by corporations, associations, and others. For details, contact the publisher at the address above.

Cover and interior book design: Claudine Mansour Design

First Edition, 2025

Paperback ISBN 978-0-9974089-0-4

Printed in the United States of America

CONTENTS

INTRODUCTION

Hello and welcome.

I'm happy you've come. I imagine you being here means something has awakened in you and is nudging you to find a new way. Perhaps what you've been doing is no longer working for you. Maybe it is no longer aligned with who you are—or maybe it never was.

You may sense that the time is now: You're ready to dive deeper into your relationship with your own self-care than you ever have before. You're ready for a deeper repatterning, a rebirthing, a coming home to yourself in a way you have never known.

If you're feeling vulnerable right now, that's okay. It is a big deal to choose to turn toward yourself in these ways. You may even feel like you don't have what it takes, or something's wrong with you because you can't seem to sustain the changes you seek.

I want you to know that there is nothing wrong with you. And you're certainly not alone.

The thing is, most of us were never taught how to care for ourselves. We were never given the "basic life skills" or what I call the "vitality fundamentals." We didn't learn how to come into an intimate understanding of all the things that nourish us, to consciously and intentionally cultivate the soil of our lives, which would have allowed us to blossom and bloom. Rather than acknowledging that we are missing these fundamentals, we unconsciously personalize our "failures," berate ourselves, and internalize the shame.

I'm here to tell you that there is another way. You *can* learn these skills. You can cultivate the necessary self-awareness, and the somatic and emotional intelligence, to sense and respond to the feedback within that is always pointing you toward what supports your vitality and away from what doesn't. This is what we'll be exploring together through the 9 Keys in *The Vitality Journal*.

The 9 Keys will guide you to examine your underlying assumptions and beliefs about health and self-care and learn what it takes to really heal your relationship with health. In other words, the keys will help you to practice a form of self-care that is actually grounded in *care*. This journey is about cultivating a fundamental orientation toward yourself that is rooted in kindness, love, and compassion, with a deep care and a fierce honoring of your unique life.

The Vitality Journal is an invitation to discover a path forward in which you will no longer need to will yourself into submission or feel like you have to manage yourself using a long checklist of self-care dos and don'ts. This is not about the quick fix. This approach is about a deeper reprogramming of your relationship to health and self-care. It's about disentangling from the patterns that aren't serving you (or anyone really) and are distracting you from what really needs tending to. It's about finding your way out from under the weight of the shame, self-judgments, and resistance—those unconscious parts that have been running the show—and see clearly the ways in which you prioritize care for others over care for yourself.

Here's the thing: *Every* choice you make every day of your life contributes to your vitality. Health is how you breathe, how you relate, how you serve—in other words, how you live. It can take time to repattern the patterns that have been there most of your life—and it takes a long-term commitment to the process. The payoff? You get to rest in the outbreath, and relax into the realization that your self-care is a life-long journey, your new center of gravity.

It is my hope that the prompts and practices within this book guide you from a place of rational understanding into a deeper, more embodied knowing, while encouraging a newfound trust in your own inner wisdom. And that you'll come into a greater understanding for yourself of what it takes to truly care for yourself, to discover what is enlivening for your body, your being. Not as a list of to-dos, but as what you do as the gardener of yourself, tending, loving, and nourishing your unique spark of life.

It is also my hope that through the words on these pages, that you will feel me right here with you. Walking the path, holding you in the complexities and all that might arise on your unique vitality journey.

HOW TO USE THIS JOURNAL

Practice, experiment, and inquire

This journal is not meant as an intellectual inquiry, but as an embodied one. Let the writing and practices you do impact all areas of your life. Live the insights, try things out, experiment, play, engage your creative, curious mind in how you move through your days. And in all of that, allow for a deep unfolding—a rebirthing, a bodily knowing, and a discovery of a new sense of self.

Take your time and make this your own

I encourage you to take your time in exploring each key and the prompts and practices within them. There is no rush here. Allow for the deeper journey and unfolding, whatever time that takes. Spend more time on the prompts, practices, and keys that are most relevant to you. And, of course, this is *your* journey, so please, trust in the pace that feels right to you.

Nature, movement, and creativity

Our inner nature and wisdom awakens in the natural world. I invite you to engage with the prompts and practices here in creative, embodied ways that resonate with you. Take the inquiry questions for walks in the woods or lie down in the grass for a few minutes before taking pen to paper. Explore your responses through drawing or other creative art forms. Let your body express the answers through authentic movement or dance. Trust your self-knowing and, again, make this your own.

Build a solid foundation

I recommend that you first work through the journal front to back (chapter by chapter). Each key builds upon the next, creating a solid foundation within you. Then circle back as often as you need to revisit the keys and prompts that are most relevant to you at a given time.

Vitality dates

While we'll be talking more about this once you get into the 9 Keys, I'd like to encourage you now to create some structures of support to keep you connected to your intentions, commitments, and regular engagement here. Start by blocking out daily or weekly time in your calendar for *The Vitality Journal*—make "vitality dates." Cozy up in your favorite armchair with a cup of tea, or take yourself to a local coffee shop; keep your journal by your bed and write in it every night before you sleep and/or first thing every morning. Find what works for you and honor the date with yourself as you would with a dear friend.

Vitality buddies

Invite a friend or loved one (a "vitality buddy"), or perhaps create a group, to join you on this journey. You might even gift a copy of this book to them as an invitation. We all thrive in relational support! Having others on the journey with you, whom you feel safe to share your vulnerabilities with, will ignite, amplify, and carry you forward. I so wish that for you and strongly encourage it. And, if no one comes to mind right now, that's fine too. Get started on your own. You can always circle back again. Also, please know that I regularly facilitate group programs based on *The Vitality Map* and *The Vitality Journal* to provide this vital relational support—go to VitalMedicine.com to sign up.

Overflow journal

As you are reflecting on the various prompts throughout this book, you may find in some instances that there isn't enough room to write, and reflect on, all that's coming through you. I'd encourage you to have another blank journal on hand for the overflow writing, so that you can write and write and write as much as you need to. This is, after all, meant to *begin* the process of catalyzing the insights—it is not the end!

Personal and professional support

As you engage with the prompts and practices in this book, a lot may get stirred up. Or you may simply benefit from the loving care and witnessing of others. Please seek out the support of friends, loved ones, and professionals, as needed.

A deeper dive

For a deeper engagement with and understanding of the 9 Keys you'll be exploring here, please read *The Vitality Map* alongside this journal— available in audiobook, ebook, or paperback versions (TheVitalityMap.com). They go together beautifully!

ADDITIONAL RESOURCES

To accompany this book, I've created a multimedia package that includes free resources to support and deepen your journey. You'll find:

+ Audio recordings of the meditations

+ PDF summaries of the 9 Keys to Deep Vitality (ready to be printed out as reminders)

+ Spreadsheets to use for awareness practices

+ And more . . .

Go to **vitalmedicine.com/vitality-journal-gifts** (or scan the QR code below) to gain access to these gifts, and look for the following symbols throughout the book to indicate when these additional resources are available to you:

🎧 *(headphones symbol)* indicates an audio recording available for download

📝 *(paper and pen symbol)* indicates a spreadsheet available for download

"You can trust
the promise of
this opening;
Unfurl yourself
into the grace of
beginning.
That is at one
with your life's
desire."

—JOHN O'DONOHUE

YOUR JOURNEY BEGINS HERE

Your vitality journey begins here, right where you are, with all the realities, roles, struggles, and history unique to you. I know from my own experience that it's nearly impossible to dive deep into new territory, to step into the unknown and give myself fully to the healing and learning that's about to happen, without getting current with myself; it's vital that I land fully in the here and now.

As you rest in the truth of your experience, and commit to being completely present to it, intentions are born. You get to feel the yearnings and desires, to touch into the visions you have for your life. It is these deeper truths that will carry you forward when you stumble, get spun around, or feel discouraged along your path.

This journey is a sacred one, a pilgrimage of sorts. In it we are cultivating a relationship with health and self-care that takes us into our depths, into a connection with the mysterious and won-drous reality of our existence, with what really matters. I'll be your guide on this pilgrimage, yet it is you who will be walking the path, *your* path. I invite you to trust in the unfolding. Trust that your way forward will reveal itself to you as you have the courage to keep opening, as you take the next step and the next and the next.

NAMING YOUR INTENTIONS & COMMITMENTS

I firmly believe in the power of clarifying and naming our intentions and commitments at the beginning of the journey. This conscious process serves to ground you and root you as you walk your unique path. It will anchor you in the larger picture of your life and clarify what this journey is about for you. The following questions will help you in preparing for your journey.

Before you begin to write, I'd encourage you to close your eyes, let your awareness drop within, and listen for that deeper inner wisdom and guidance.

✦ What intentions do you have for embarking on this journey?

✦ What are you yearning to receive and learn?

✦ What are you willing to give to this experience?

✦ What potential obstacles do you foresee in implementing the life changes you seek?

✦ Who do you know who could sincerely and consistently support you as you embark on this transformative healing path?

Once you have finished writing your answers, I invite you to share them with someone you trust, someone who will hold the sacredness and vulnerability of this journey with you. By having someone you trust listen to you declare your intentions and commitments out loud—without judgment—it can often be easier to connect with those intentions and commitments, and to truly embody them. They can become more real. You may even want to invite a friend or loved one along with you on this journey— someone ready and eager to dive deep in the same ways that you are. Together, you can create an ongoing path of mutual sharing, learning, growing, and healing.

WHAT'S TO COME

Now that you've had a chance to reflect and explore your intentions for your journey, I wanted to give you a glimpse of what's to come.

These are the 9 Keys to Deep Vitality that you'll be engaging with in the rest of the journal. As you read the title of each key below, pause for a moment and notice what's surfacing for you. How and where does each one land in your body? What emotional qualities arise for you? What associations do you immediately have? Jot down your reflections below.

Here you are now at the threshold of your journey. In naming your intentions and commitments, you have put a stake in the ground, declaring your willingness to open, heal, learn, and evolve. There is such potency in that!

I want to honor the courage it takes to begin this journey, to explore the prompts and practices here, to open to what emerges and arises, to be with the hard truths and move into the unknown. You've already had a taste of what awaits you at the foundational levels of your being. Now you have the opportunity to explore how you move through life and how you care for yourself along the way. You are about to step onto the path of liberating your own well-being. And, in the spirit of pilgrimage, you will discover, as I have, that health is not a destination—it *is* the journey.

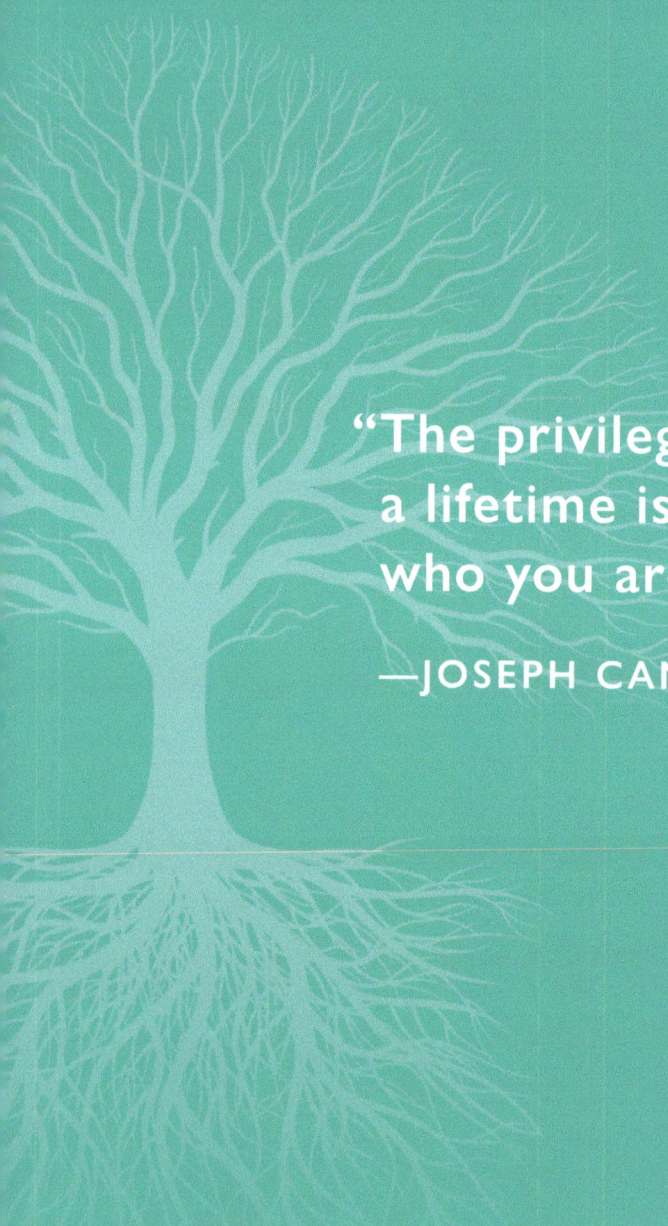

"The privilege of a lifetime is being who you are."

—JOSEPH CAMPBELL

HONORING YOUR UNIQUE LIFE

The first of the nine keys, Honoring Your Unique Life, is at the root of this whole journey. It is about waking up to the precious gift and miracle of being alive as *you*. You are the only you there is and will ever be, an utterly unique expression of life. By cultivating an ongoing awareness of the fleeting nature of life and being present to your mortality, you can begin to connect with the innate responsibility you have to consciously steward and care for your life.

You may have experienced this in sweet moments of connection, such as holding a newborn baby in your arms, experiencing a glorious sunrise, having a heart-to-heart conversation with someone you love, or even tending to someone who is dying. Afterwards, you vow to never again take this extraordinary life for granted. And then, you do. We all do. The joy, the wonder, even the grief fades, and we go back to sleep. We drift from the sacredness of our lives, from the reverence our bodies deserve. What would it take to come to know these sacred moments more regularly, as a day-to-day embodied experience? How might it feel to move through your life with that wonder and reverence as your center of gravity?

Through rooting your self-care in reverence and gratitude for this life, you can embrace a sense of authorship. There's no need to wait for a moment of inspiring beauty or an unexpected tragedy to awaken to this. You can access it right now. Because here's the thing: No one else is here to do it for you. Each of us must do it for ourselves; we are born into this "job," to serve and honor our unique life expression. This is the core of our innate responsibility in life—and it is our privilege and honor.

COMING HOME TO YOUR BODY

The following visualization invites you to feel what it means to be you, to be fully alive in this unique body. As you enter into this meditation, keep in mind the words of the activist Joanna Macy, who writes, "To participate in the dance of life with senses to perceive it, lungs that breathe it, organs that draw nourishment from it—is a wonder beyond words."[1]

🎧 Imagine you are meeting your body for the very first time. Close your eyes, conjuring the curious spirit of a young child, and notice the subtle sensations that tell you you're alive in this moment. What are you noticing in your physical body? See if you can visualize the life-energy coursing through you—breathing you, pumping blood through your veins. What does it feel like to be breathed?

Now notice your senses—hearing, seeing, smelling, tasting, and touching. What is surfacing for you? What thoughts are floating through your awareness? What emotions are you feeling?

And finally, pause and let your awareness move into the

stillness that exists beneath all of the layers of who you are. Take a moment to reflect on the astonishing reality that you are alive, in a body, and are able to be consciously aware of all of this. As you slowly open your eyes, take some time to receive what arose for you in coming home to yourself in this way, then jot down some insights here.

YOU ARE UNIQUE

You are the only you there is and will ever be. Ever. Not only is it a miracle that any of us are alive, in a body and conscious of it, but each of us looks out through eyes that only we can see through, has thoughts only we think, has a sense of "me" that no one else can ever experience. We're all expressions of the same life-energy, and yet we are each utterly unique.

I love how Martha Graham speaks to this in another way:

> There is a vitality, a life force, an energy, a quickening, that is translated through you into action, and because there is only one of you in all time, this expression is unique. And if you block it, it will never exist through any other medium and will be lost. The world will not have it. It is not your business to determine how good

it is nor how valuable nor how it compares with other expressions. It is your business to keep it yours clearly and directly, to keep the channel open.[2]

Take some time to reflect on all that arises for you as you sit with these sentiments.

TAKING RESPONSIBILITY

For many people, responsibility can be a bit of a loaded word, in that gotta-get-it-right, can't-mess-up kind of way. Key #1 explores how to come into a new relationship with self-responsibility. Before we go there, it is important to see with clear eyes, to get honest with yourself about how you currently take responsibility for your own well-being.

First, write down the word "responsibility." You might even say it out loud a few times.

Next, take a few minutes and make a stream-of-consciousness list of all of the knee-jerk feelings, associations, and reactions you have when you see and hear the word "responsibility" in relation to your health and self-care. If there are parts of you that are feeling activated by this inquiry, pause and check in with them. What visceral reactions are surfacing? What emotions want to be acknowledged? Listen with tenderness and patience, writing down anything that comes up in this inquiry.

REBELLIOUS TEENAGER OR STRICT PARENT?

When it comes to taking responsibility for our self-care, many of us have a combination of parts that can sound either a lot like a Strict parent or a Rebellious Teenager. The Strict Parent tells us in no uncertain terms about all the things we are *supposed to be doing* to take responsibility for our health, right now and in this particular way. The Rebellious Teenager avoids it all, not wanting to take responsibility for anything. Look back at the writing you just did to see which of those parts might be especially loud for you.

In general, how do you experience those two voices playing out in you? When do they show up? Do you predominantly identify with one more than the other, or do they cycle back and forth?

CHECKING IN

Pause now and check in with yourself. You may want to close your eyes or soften your gaze, and take a moment to feel your feet on the ground. Consciously connect with your breath, filling your abdomen and gently expanding your diaphragm with each in-breath. Gently invite the pace of your breathing to slow and your attention to open outward through your senses. Bring a big dose of gentle compassion and gratitude to those parts of you you've just connected with (e.g., the inner Strict Parent and the Rebellious Teenager), feeling your capacity to simply be with them, accepting them just as they are, without judgment.

YOUR SECRET SUPERPOWER: MAMA BEAR LOVE

Feeling overwhelmed by a sense of self-responsibility often means that we've disconnected from gratitude and reverence for what the poet Mary Oliver calls our "one wild and precious life."[3] What if you could shift from seeing self-care as a burden to viewing it as a privilege and an act of self-love and compassion, a way of wrapping your arms around yourself?

When I think of such a warm, loving embrace, I think about a mama bear with her cubs. Picture that for a moment. What qualities does she possess? How does she show up for and tend to her cubs? How does she respond when something threatens the well-being of her little ones?

Imagine cultivating a quality of presence akin to the fierce love of a mama bear. Think of someone you love like that—your child, a pet. Feel it fully in your body the way that mama-bear love shows up—the loyalty, the protectiveness, the unwavering devotion to the welfare of those she loves, the tender, sweet care combined with a no-nonsense fierceness and strength; take a little extra time to feel those mama-bear hugs—they're the best!

Describe how that feels in your body, heart, and being.

Now, turn that inner Mama Bear love toward yourself. Feel her embrace. Feel how she has your back, how she'll stand in the fire for you, do what it takes to hold *your* welfare at the center of her awareness. Feel her devotion to nourishing your well-being, on all levels, to supporting your growth and evolution.

Describe what has arisen in this imagining? How does it feel to be embraced so unconditionally? So fiercely? Give yourself permission to not censor yourself here.

And now recognize that she, your inner Mama Bear, is *you*, your essence, the core of your being. How does it feel to embrace the realization that you alone are responsible for your "wild and precious life"? From your inner Mama Bear voice, what does it mean to honor that unique life?

Pause and check in with yourself. Sometimes when we tune into this kind of love, it can bring up grief for the ways we were so imperfectly loved when we were young, or the ways in which we have not been able to love ourselves. Move slowly and gently through these feelings. How might you express them in writing, by moving your body, and through your voice?

YOU ARE MORTAL

To fully and lovingly accept responsibility for your life means confronting and being in direct relationship with your own mortality. Sometimes that can happen after a troubling diagnosis, a near-death experience, or even reading the news about the death of a child in a freak accident. Regardless of how it happens, it can leave us with the realization of how fleeting and unpredictable life really is. And with that often comes a willingness to prioritize what really matters, to be present to the extraordinariness of our life. Naturally, none of us knows how long we are going to be here. We simply don't.

Think of a time when you've had to confront your own mortality or grieve the death of someone close to you. What happened inside you in the aftermath of these experiences? What awoke in you? What realizations did you have about your life? How did your perspectives shift?

As you sit with these memories and realizations, what feels most relevant and important to remind yourself of at this moment in your life?

How might being in a direct relationship with your own mortality support you in your life moving forward?

Years ago, I had a daily practice of asking myself, "If I were to die today, would I feel complete?" It brought a potency of awareness to my daily life, and catalyzed a lot of actions: reaching out to loved ones, listening with more attunement to my intuition and callings, taking more risks, and not waiting to create the life that aligns with my Yes! Is there a similar question that you can embrace as a practice?

Take a look in the mirror and say to yourself (or even out loud) right now: "I am fucking alive! I get to be alive right now!" How did that feel?

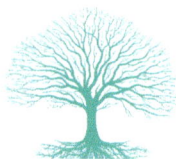

> *"An awareness of one's mortality can lead you to wake up and live an authentic, meaningful life."*[4] —Bernie Siegel, MD

GARDENING YOURSELF

Imagine that you are a gardener, with a backyard garden plot. In the spring, you head out and prepare your beds for planting. You dig up the weeds and the old mulch, fork the soil, add compost, and plant some seeds. You meticulously tend to those seeds—watering them and waiting for that moment when little seedlings push their way up through the soil. Turning your attention to those seedlings, you pull the weeds from around them and offer extra nutrients when necessary. Over time, those seedlings lengthen and change form; they blossom and bear fruits.

As the gardener you are not in charge of guiding the unique form and expression the plant takes. The life-force within the plant does that. You are, however, in charge of showing up, tending to the plant, paying attention and staying aware of it day after day. You must provide what the plant needs in support of its evolution.

Pause for a moment to consider this: The life-force within the seed you planted that enables it to germinate, emerge, grow, blossom, and bloom into its unique expression, is the *same vital energy that is in you*. Now try on the orientation that you are simply the gardener of yourself, of the life-energy infusing your particular body and being. Your core responsibility is to tend to this life each and every day. You are here to serve life in this unique expression that you are.

In this moment, through the lens of being the gardener of yourself, answer the following questions, knowing that we will circle back to these inquiries in various ways in the subsequent chapters:

What nourishes and supports your unique "body-being"? What does it need to become and remain as vibrant and alive as it can be?

What might be currently blocking your ability to receive the nourishment you need? What might need to be weeded from your garden bed?

In what contexts are you planted (e.g., home, location, environment, work, social circles)? How do each of these contexts support (or hinder) your unique constitution, needs, and being? What other contexts might you plant yourself in that would support your well-being, emergence, and growth?

Do you have the room you need to stretch, grow, emerge, follow your impulses, and reach for the sun without limit? What might allow for your life-energy to feel free to fully express itself?

As you allow all of that to percolate in your consciousness, take another moment to pause. Invite your awareness into your body, feeling that innate life-energy infusing every cell of your being. Find your feet. Feel the support beneath you.

TAKEAWAYS

✦ In your own words, describe what Key #1 means to you.

✦ What are three things you are taking away from this exploration with Key #1?

✦ What intentions do you have for the coming days, including any holding/support you may want to seek out.

BRINGING IT ALL TOGETHER

Key #1—Honoring Your Unique Life is about shifting out of an unconscious attitude of taking life for granted. It's about healing the orientation so many of us have around self-responsibility in relation to our health and self-care, one in which we might will ourselves into submission, then rebel against that, finding ourselves in a boom-and-bust cycle.

Instead, we can wake up to the preciousness of life, embrace our inner Mama Bear and welcome being the gardener of ourselves. We are each here to become more of who we are through a mindset of reverence, gratitude, and honoring, and by tending to our needs, nourishing our bodies, beings, and our innate unfolding and expression.

We'll circle back to this key often. Don't be surprised if your explorations thus far have felt significant, not so much from an intellectual standpoint, but from a deeper repatterning that will allow you to embody a new center of gravity. I encourage you to trust in the process you are in and be open to whatever is being stirred within you. It is not uncommon for grief to arise. Go slow. Be gentle with yourself and with the parts within that may get activated. And remember this key at its root is about turning toward yourself with kindness, grace, love, and a deep honoring of your unique life.

"If we can't embrace the whole of who we are—embrace it with transformative love—we'll imprison the creative energies hidden in our own shadows and be unable to engage creatively with the world's complex mix of shadow and light."

—PARKER PALMER

FACING AND EMBRACING YOUR SHADOWS

In *Key #1—Honoring Your Unique Life,* you may have experienced moments of sweet connection, felt reverence for your own precious life, and even a sense of self-responsibility akin to a mother's love. You may have also discovered that it's one thing to get a taste of this and quite another to actually live it, day to day. Maybe you've noticed that you can't seem to sustain the changes you began putting in place, or you're having trouble prioritizing what matters most to you. It's easy to conclude: *I should know better. There must be something wrong with me. I don't have the discipline it takes.*

These unhelpful, judgmental thoughts can bring up so much shame. If this is your experience, know that you're not alone. Many of us find our health and self-care journey a challenge to navigate. Why? Because we can't avoid also discovering our shadows, which psychologist Carl Jung describes as the parts of ourselves that run the show behind the scenes, the parts we have unconsciously rejected, disowned, or repressed. That's why *Key #2—Facing & Embracing Your Shadows* is such an essential part of your journey into deep personal healing.

It can take a lot of your life-energy to pretend to be something you're not. Those disowned parts of yourself are like a hole in the bucket, draining your life-energy, zapping your vitality.

When you can consciously shine light on your shadow parts, shedding and releasing all the layers of armor you've built up around them, accepting all of who you are, it's like breaking out of prison. You naturally blossom and thrive; you have the capacity to receive what nourishes you and to make choices that are in alignment with what brings you fully alive. But how do you get there? How do you even begin? By first naming and facing your shadows—we can't heal what we don't acknowledge—and then welcoming them into the light, accepting and embracing them without judgment.

FACING YOUR SHADOWS

It's not always easy to identify our shadows—they're hidden for a reason! Even when we commit to doing the work, our shadows can often seem more obvious to others than they are to us. They might not know the roots or stories attached to our shadows, but they can see them at play in ways we can't, until we start to consciously explore them. While the prompts in this chapter are geared toward a solo discovery process, please keep in mind that we often need others in these shadowy realms to help us see what we can't see on our own.

Before you dive in, here are a few reminders: You're moving into tender territory. Be patient, take your time, and be gentle with yourself. And when you're ready, please root yourself here in this orientation: As the shadow parts come into light you turn toward them with empathy, compassion, and love, just as you would do for a friend who is in pain. You listen to them with curiosity, open to hear and be with them in their suffering, to understand the perspectives they bring. You offer them a seat at the table and welcome them home, with a big Mama Bear hug. And remember, sometimes what gets in your way—those shadow parts—may also be what shows you the way. I invite you to stay open to that possibility.

Avoidance and self-sabotage

The ways in which we subtly (or not so subtly) ignore our needs, numb out, or cause harm to ourselves is all ripe territory to explore the shadows at play. Consider the following questions:

How do you block your own thriving?

What avoidance patterns are you aware of in relation to your self-care? What examples come to mind when you consider how you might be sabotaging your own attempts at caring for your well-being? Are there behaviors or habits you're engaging in that make you feel unwell?

When do these patterns of avoidance and self-sabotage flare up for you? Do they happen after feeling certain strong emotions? Or after spending time with a particular person? Perhaps after a long day at work? Describe any correlations that you discover.

Resistance

When we feel resistance, it can be pretty clear that shadows are at play. It's as though the role of resistance is to distract us from facing our shadows. But what if, paradoxically, resistance is really a signal to us to pay attention? What if we could use resistance to help us to accept our shadows instead of turning away from them? Bring them into the light instead of keeping them in the dark? What if our resistance becomes a crucial guide along our path to freedom and wholeness?

Author Steven Pressfield says it so well:

> Most of us have two lives. The life we live, and the unlived life within us. Between the two stands Resistance . . . We can navigate by Resistance, letting it guide us to that calling or action that we must follow before all others. Rule of thumb: The more important a call or action is to our soul's evolution, the more Resistance we will feel toward pursuing it.[5]

✦ What does resistance look like for you?

✦ How and when does it show up in your life?

✦ What does it feel like in your body?

✦ What behaviors emerge in response to resistance?

Reactions to other people

Think back on a time you had a strong, visceral reaction to something someone said or did. You may even have wondered what could have triggered a reaction like that. When that happens, it's often an indication that you are seeing in them aspects of yourself you have long buried or disowned. Since it's way easier to see things in others that we can't see in ourselves, noticing such reactions can be a doorway into your own shadow parts.

What are some of the strong reactions you have had recently to other people?

See if you can identify any qualities in other people that you really dislike, or maybe even are repulsed by. What are they? How do they make you feel? What happens in you when you're around them?

Have you had any recent conflicts where you were sure that you were "right"? Where the other person's perspective or stance was something you felt you could never adopt?

Do you put anyone up on a pedestal? Who and what qualities do they possess that you admire?

Now pause for a moment to reconnect with your body and breath. For each question you answered, consider if any of the perspectives or qualities that repulsed, irritated, or offended you, or evoked a sense of envy or admiration, are parts that may also live within you.

Take your time with this—it can bring up a lot and be challenging as you confront and let go of ideas you have had about yourself while also expanding your sense of self.

Breaking the shame spiral

This process of bringing things out into the light can create a big layer of shame and self-judgment. You might feel that you are stuck or that you are not okay as you are. You might be convinced that something must be wrong with you and that all of these new revelations should remain hidden. Where there is shame, there are shadows.

✦ What are the points of the most shame for you in your health and self-care journey?

✦ How does it feel now to name them?

✦ Have you shared them with anyone before? If so, how did that feel?

✦ What is most uncomfortable for you about these aspects of yourself?

✦ What feels most embarrassing? What feels most vulnerable?

✦ What's your sense of what is underneath the shame? What feeds it?

✦ How does the shame you feel impact your motivation to create change?

Golden shadows

Shadows are not all connected to the parts of ourselves we deem negative or unacceptable. We also have "golden" shadows, as Jung called them. We have strengths, creativity, and brilliance that we have unconsciously blocked, which keeps us from shining in the world. Think of your golden shadow as your "repressed greatness," or hidden talents you may be too afraid or insecure to reveal. Perhaps you love to sing and have even been told you have a lovely voice, but for myriad reasons, you can't seem to make yourself sing in front of anyone. Or you've been writing poetry for years, but the idea of sharing it with others fills you with dread.

Marianne Williamson captures this phenomenon in one of her famous quotations: "Our deepest fear is not that we are inadequate. Our deepest fear is that we are powerful beyond measure.

It is our light, not our darkness, that most frightens us."[6] Facing and embracing your golden shadows brings these untapped or suppressed aspects of ourselves out into the light.

Pause here for a moment to let that in. You likely have golden shadows at play, and their influence can be even more powerful than the parts you would typically identify as shadows. They are born from our childhood woundings, trauma, what was modeled for us, who we were told we could be, the lack of safety we have felt to authentically express ourselves, and more.

✦ Where might you have a golden shadow at play? How do you dim your brilliance? In what ways do you subdue or suppress the expression of your gifts, your unique genius?

✦ What are you afraid might be revealed if you bring the shadows to the surface and allow yourself to thrive?

✦ What do you tell yourself would happen if you let yourself truly shine and be seen in all your greatness?

✦ What might be preventing those golden parts of you from coming to the surface and shining brightly?

CHECKING IN

Pause for a moment and check in with yourself. You might like to take yourself outside, feel your feet on the ground, breathe in the fresh air. What are you feeling right now—in your body, emotionally, in your psyche, spiritually. Take some time to journal and reflect. We have been touching into so much! How can you turn toward yourself with more kindness in this moment?

What do you need right now? Don't be surprised if you aren't really sure. The degree of shadow that swirls with our shame and the raw vulnerability that surfaces can keep us from even being able to identify our needs.

Perhaps there's something else on the periphery, something so central to what's going on for you that you have overlooked it.

It might be something that you haven't named here that might be enmeshed with so much protection around it that you couldn't even access it before.

Try sitting softly and gently with yourself with an openness and willingness to be with your truth, whatever it may be.

WORKING WITH THE SHADOW PARTS

We've been exploring our shadows as different parts of ourselves. Some we meet with resistance and shame, while others—those golden ones—we can meet with surprise and curiosity. So far, we've been excavating and touching into these parts; now let's explore them more explicitly.

I like to think of working with our shadow parts as akin to inviting those parts to come out of the darkness and have a seat at our inner round table. There we can talk, listen with empathy and curiosity, and create a direct relationship with them—*in the light.*

We start with those parts that are already vocal, that have a lot to say. What they say may be painful and difficult to hear. These are the really loud voices inside of us; those that have brought their own megaphones to shout into!

What are some of your loud habitual parts, the familiar disruptive voices in your head? Some common ones are the Critic, Self-judger, Perfectionist, Rebellious Teenager, Strict Parent.

What do they have to say?

What might you name them?

Can you think of a habitual persona (the "you") that you present to the world? What vulnerabilities or deeper truths might you be unconsciously protecting by hiding behind the mask of your persona (e.g., smiling when you are feeling upset, appearing calm and confident when you are nervous)? What shadow parts might be hidden from view?

Inviting more parts to the table

Here's the thing: Once you've invited the loud ones to the table, you can now invite the rest of the voices to the table. There is always room for any and all parts of yourself. Sometimes they simply show up on their own, but sometimes they are so quiet, or have been in the shadows for so long, that they need an empathic presence, and the promise of deep listening so they can share what they need to share. In this way, we can broaden how we hold ourselves on our journey, to recognize myriad perspectives within.

Imagine the different kinds of perspectives and guidance you might open to if more parts joined you at the table.

What are some inner voices that have your back, that want to help you thrive in life?

What are other ones you might invite (let your creativity go wild here . . . the inner Nurturer, the Wise Grandmother, the inner Mama Bear, your Loyal Friend, your inner Rockstar!)?

EMBRACING YOUR SHADOWS

After seeing our shadow parts directly, bringing them into the light, then there is the embrace. We cultivate a direct relationship with them; we show up with a compassionate and curious presence, accepting and being with all of who they are. The healing comes in the embrace. The parts soften when they are held in love. They evolve and transform, integrating into our sense of wholeness, the truth of who we are. And we come home more fully to ourselves as the parts emerging from the shadows are given a seat at the table.

If you are exploring your shadows on your own, you can cultivate this kind of relationship with each part, through journaling. Here's how: (Warning: This might feel silly and weird to you, but it works! Experiment and see for yourself.)

1. **Choose the part** you'd like to connect with. If you're not sure how to choose, review your answers to the journaling prompts above and see if any feel especially activated in you at this particular moment in time. It may help to attach a gender and a name to your part; or keep it gender neutral like I have here.

2. **Ground and center** in whatever ways works for you. You might connect with your feet, feeling the support beneath you. And follow your breath as it cycles in and out. Open to your senses—what you are seeing, hearing, feeling, tasting, smelling. Take your time with this until you feel very present to this moment.

3. **Drop into your inner Mama Bear** and imagine turning toward this shadow part as you would a friend who is suffering or going through a lot. You are not there to fix or change it in any way, but to simply show up with a loving presence: Listen with empathy and compassion. Let it know that you are here for it and that it is no longer alone. Bring your curiosity and openness—approach this part as if you have never met it before. (If you are struggling to do this, or find yourself identifying as the part, return to step 2).

4. **Connect fully** with this part until you have a real felt sense of it—a feeling in your body, an image, a voice in your head. And then have a conversation with your part here. Write

down both your questions and reflections as well as its answers. Let go of needing to know; truly listen for what comes through when you inquire. Again, imagine that you are meeting your part for the first time. You might ask it about how it's feeling, what it sees as its job, how it's trying to help you. Ask your part what it most wants you to know about it. Suspend your inner skeptic, use your intuition here.

5. **Practice conscious listening** and reflect back to your part what you are hearing. Let it feel seen and understood and remind it that you are there for it. Let it know you appreciate all it's been doing and all it's gone through. You are cultivating a relationship of trust. And have patience, as it can take a while sometimes for parts that have been disowned to open and share. You can also sit with your part in silence, simply letting it know you are there.

6. **Thank the part.** To close your conversations, let your part know how much connecting with it matters; tell it you care and that you'll be back.

7. **Repeat regularly** with individual parts until they might transform and no longer need that regular contact. And try it out with other parts. This is an ongoing practice of shadow integration that is available to you.

And stay attuned to when you might need to bring professional support on board to help with this integration.

TAKEAWAYS

✦ In your own words, describe what Key #2 means to you.

✦ What are three things you are taking away from this exploration with Key #2?

✦ What intentions do you have for the coming days, including any holding/support you may want to seek out?

BRINGING IT ALL TOGETHER

As we are wrapping up this key, I want to emphasize a few things. First, we all have shadows—every one of us—parts operating in our unconscious. You didn't do anything wrong and there is nothing wrong with you. So much of what is in our shadows has been passed down through generations to us. So, in turning toward them, and bringing them into the light, you are healing not only yourself but shifting generational patterns.

Second, we need each other here in the shadowy realms. The reflections of others help us to see what we can't see on our own, to learn how to compassionately love the parts of ourselves that we may have consciously or unconsciously rejected. And yet, having discernment about who you share with and how you share is essential; it's important that you feel safe and compassionately held in revealing your hurt parts, your vulnerabilities, and your shame.

And as you turn toward the parts that have been disowned, that have been down in the deep dark basement, a lot may move through you—grief, anger, painful memories. Be gentle with yourself. Take your time. Bring lots of compassion and love. And *please*, do not hesitate to reach out for personal and professional support here.

"Not biology,
but ignorance
of ourselves,
has been the
key to our
powerlessness."

—ADRIENNE RICH

STRENGTHENING YOUR SELF-AWARENESS MUSCLES

How often have you felt spun around by the latest health fad? The newest research that seems to refute the latest and greatest discovery you read about only a few months before? How do you know what's true and what's hype? It all sounds plausible. To add to your confusion, what about all the health advice you get from people in your life (whether you ask for it or not)—your hairstylist, your mom, your colleagues, your best friend, even the guy at the coffee shop. Everyone thinks they know what you should be doing to take care of yourself. Of course, they rarely agree with one another. It can feel a bit crazymaking, right?

When you listen to these authorities (including your doctors), you run the risk of tuning out the one expert you need to be listening to first and foremost: *You.* You are the only one who can read the feedback that comes directly from your body-being *in real time*—feedback that can point the way toward better health, and give you the information you need to begin to move from floundering to flourishing.

Let me repeat that: *No one else but you can receive the feedback you need from your body and your being.*

Key #3—Strengthening Your Self-Awareness Muscles is all about becoming a conscious explorer of yourself and developing empowered self-intimacy. And through this process, you can come to own your authority and develop a clear trust in your self-knowing.

DON'T HOLD BACK

Have you ever left a doctor's office and felt disempowered, confused, and overwhelmed by the prognosis you received or the medications you were prescribed? Then you know what it feels like to look for and rely on answers outside of yourself that supposedly direct your healthcare choices, rather than starting from within.

Think back to a time when you gave someone else the power to diagnose and treat you even when you weren't sure about their conclusion. How did it feel to outsource that decision? What did you give away? How did that feel in your body? And how did it impact your confidence and self-trust? Go ahead. Let. It. Rip. Don't hold back. This is the beginning of seeing with clear eyes the terrain you have traversed and expanding your self-awareness. We have to start exactly where we are.

THE ANSWERS LIE WITHIN

The feedback from your body-being has always been there—your whole life—even though you may not have been aware of it. Like a friendly whisper in your ear, the feedback's voice usually starts out very soft and gentle. And then, if you don't seem to hear it— either because you haven't yet learned how to pay attention to it or there's something in your shadow self that won't allow you to engage with it—the feedback will get louder, and Louder, and LOUDER, until you feel like you've run into a proverbial brick wall. Turns out the only way around or over the wall is to pause, listen to what your body-being is trying to tell you, and respond accordingly.

Sometimes it's not until we look back on a health scare or other challenge that we realize the whispers and nudges we were receiving from inside our bodies were in fact spot on. Indeed, having the benefit of hindsight can help us understand the feedback we were receiving all along. Once you learn the language of your internal feedback, as you will with this key, you'll begin to hear it when it's a soft and loving nudge, rather than waiting for a forceful smack over the head.

Describe a time when, in hindsight, you realized you missed some critical cues from your internal feedback, and then it was too late. What were those whispers you missed? What got you to pay attention?

What inklings of feedback might be there for you right now? Can you tune into them when they are still quiet and gentle? Is there feedback for you that is getting louder and more insistent?

READING THE FEEDBACK SIGNALS

Many of us have become more self-aware in areas other than those involving our health—through spiritual practices, building conscious relationships, working to heal past traumas, or being in therapy. But we seem to stop short when it comes to our health. We simply haven't learned the language that allows us to ask for the information we need, so we can too easily misinterpret what the body is telling us. The following meditation and the questions afterward are the first steps toward strengthening your self-awareness muscles. Before getting started, here are a few things to remember:

1. **Cultivate a beginner's mind.** Each time you enter into self-inquiry, you're going to have a brand-new experience. So start right where you are. Stay open and curious—observe and learn.

2. **Take your time.** Slowing down is an essential step toward building a strong foundation for your vitality and self-care for the rest of your life. Linger in places that call to you.

3. **Simply observe.** You'll likely want to act on what you've discovered. Instead, wait. Allow your awareness to continue to expand and your muscles of self-observation to strengthen, then the action you do take will be more aligned with the realities of your life and your unique body-being. The next key, Key #4, is all about taking action. For now, simply observe and practice patience.

4. **Repeat the practice often**. As you strengthen your awareness muscles, you begin to understand the nuances of what you are experiencing. This allows you to become more sensitive and fine-tuned in your capacity to receive the feedback that is there.

PRACTICING SELF-AWARENESS

🎧 Find a comfortable upright position in which you can relax for several minutes. Close your eyes or soften your gaze as you explore the following. Pause to reflect in writing as you go or wait until the end. Your choice.

Move your attention into your body, as though you are discovering it for the first time. How does it feel to be in a body, *your* body? What do you notice right away? Where is your attention drawn?

What area of your body feels the most relaxed? Linger there for a moment. Notice a part of your body that feels tense or uncomfortable. Does it change or stay the same when you bring your awareness there? Describe what you notice and any judgments or reactions you are having.

Bring awareness to your feelings. What emotions are arising? Where do you sense those feelings in your body? What is the quality of those sensations? What story or memory surfaces as you become aware of the feelings?

Check in with yourself: What is your energetic state (e.g., sluggish, impatient, settled, nervous)? Get specific in describing your assessment. Consider how your current feelings and experiences in your body, your mind, and your emotions relate to your energetic state. Now see if you are able to drop into a deeper quality of presence that includes a spiritual orientation or consciousness. What do you notice now?

Expand your awareness outwardly. Notice what you're picking up on in your environment right now (e.g., temperature, sounds, smells, tastes, textures, sights). And then notice how your body and being respond to those stimuli. What feels nourishing and what does not? Any preferences or aversions?

As you emerge from this meditative practice, take some time to reflect on all that you noticed. What felt familiar? What felt new or unfamiliar? What was hard for you to even feel or acknowledge?

FLEXING YOUR SELF-AWARENESS MUSCLES

In service to the deep listening and reflecting you've been doing in meditation, here are some ways to expand your awareness into different areas of your life. First, a caveat. Don't feel you must "master" every area listed below. These categories are signposts on your vitality map. Think of them as examples to seed your awareness and help you discover what's relevant to you right now. At each location you can focus in and dive as deep as you choose. You may want to start with those areas you feel are the most challenging for your self-care: Diet? Sleep? Intimacy? Elimination? Then consider what kind of data feedback you're looking for.

Digestion, nutrition, and eating

Full Disclosure: I am not a fan of dieting or the myriad ways our culture fat-shames us into an unhealthy and often complicated relationship with food. This has nothing to do with any of that! Quite the opposite. This is about developing an attentive and conscious relationship with the foods you eat.

Questions to consider: What foods are comforting for you? What foods seem to make you come alive? What foods make you feel tired and deadened? How present are you when you're eating? How quickly or slowly are you consuming your food? Notice how that may affect the way you feel afterward or the quality of your digestion. Any gas? Any discomfort?

What in this topic are you curious to explore more and why?

Breathing

Paying attention to your breathing can give you important clues into how you're feeling physically, mentally and emotionally.

Questions to consider: What parts of you move as you breathe in and out? Which feels easier—the inhalation or exhalation? Are you breathing quickly or slowly? Long breaths or short? Does your breathing feel restricted or open? Shallow or deep? How does your breath change when you feel stressed or calm? Happy or worried? How does playing around with the pace and depth of your breath affect how you are feeling?

What in this topic are you curious to explore and why?

Sleep

We spend about one-third of our lives sleeping, and it is not idle time. So much repair, healing, and recovery happens, along with hormone regulation, memory consolidation, immune system processes, and more.

Questions to consider: What is the quality of your sleep? Do you wake up rested or sluggish? How does your ability to roll with things change when you don't get enough sleep? What evening and bedtime routines do you have? If you are not feeling rejuvenated from your sleep, what are some behavior patterns you notice throughout your day or into the evening that might be impacting the quality of your sleep, including stimulating substances or activities.

What in this topic are you curious to explore and why?

Elimination pathways

Strengthening your physical awareness of your elimination pathways means taking note of the quality, odor, appearance, and quantity of what your body is releasing. It also means how your body-being moves through thoughts and emotions before they get stuck and cause illness.

Questions to consider: How much water are you drinking? How often do you pee and what color is it? How much do you sweat? What does your breath smell like? How often do you poop? What does it look like or smell like? How is your poop affected by what you eat? What does it feel like in your body when strong emotions or thoughts are asking to be released? What symptoms arise? What happens for you when they get stuck on repeat?

What in this topic are you curious to explore and why?

Thoughts and emotions

Everything you feel, everything you think about is mirrored in your body. A stressful day can show up in your facial expressions, the tone of your voice, and even your posture. Sometimes those connections are easy to notice, but other times, not so much.

Questions to consider: Bring a stressful situation to mind. How does thinking about it affect your body? What about a joyful moment. Did your posture or facial expression change? Consciously play around with your body, shifting positions, and see what might change. If you find yourself in a stress reaction, notice all of the physical symptoms of that (e.g., heart rate, perspiration, breath rate and quality, temperature in your extremities).

What in this topic are you curious to explore and why?

Relaxation and play

How often do you indulge in unstructured time that is purely for your enjoyment? If you're like so many of us, the fun stuff—the time spent daydreaming, the activities that bring us joy—is what gets pushed to the side when other aspects of life demand our attention.

Questions to consider: What does play look like for you? What do you find deeply restorative? Who and/or what in your life inspires heartfelt laughter and open-hearted joy? What helps your nervous system to slow down and truly relax?

What in this topic are you curious to explore and why?

Movement and flexibility

Sometimes it can be hard to stop what you're doing and move your body. And your body may respond loudly with aches and pains and stiff joints.

Questions to consider: What gets you moving during your day? What types of movement do you enjoy? What comes naturally to your body? What activities feel unpleasant or even impossible? How do different positions—standing, sitting, bending over your computer, doing something physically demanding—impact your body and your state of being? How does your body respond to everyday movements, such as walking up or down stairs or around the block, bending down to lift things, carrying your child, running for the bus?

What in this topic are you curious to explore and why?

Sexuality

It's interesting how difficult it can be to talk openly about our sexual energy, which really is synonymous with our life-energy, our innate creative force.

Questions to consider: Whether it is with yourself and/or a partner, how open are you to experiencing sensual and sexual pleasure these days? Does it feel enlivening or is there a sense of avoidance or resistance? How comfortable are you with your sexuality? With sensual touch? If you are engaging in sexual activity with yourself or a partner, how do you feel before, during, and after? Is there anything else you want or need to acknowledge in your relationship with your sexuality?

What in this topic are you curious to explore and why?

Attention

Even though recent studies have proven that multitasking increases stress levels, negatively impacts creativity, and leads to burnout, we are still culturally encouraged to take pride in our ability to juggle multiple tasks. It's a hard habit to break.

Questions to consider: What are some of the surprising ways you multitask in your life? How does technology impact where your attention goes at any given moment? How does it feel when you are engaging in three different things at once? How does it feel when you step away from your phone for a couple of hours? When you put everything aside and head out into nature? What arises for you if you simply sit quietly with yourself for a while?

What in this topic are you *curious* to explore and why?

CHECKING IN

At this point in your process, it is important to pause and take a few healing, grounding breaths. Perhaps take yourself for a walk outside or stand up and shake out your body. How is all this landing so far for you? Notice if it's possible for you to hold yourself a bit more gently and lovingly as you move forward into this new territory.

CHOOSING WHERE TO START

There are myriad ways that you can begin to expand and deepen your self-awareness, as you probably noticed when you engaged with the various categories above. You can't focus on everything all at once (that's crazymaking!). Start with the areas that feel particularly relevant at this time in your life or areas that are the most challenging right now in relation to your self-care. And then choose what kind of information would be most helpful to you.

Describe the intentions for your awareness practice here in detail. What will you be observing? How will you be physically tracking or reflecting upon your learning? What tools do you have on hand (e.g., calendar reminders, Post-it notes, task app on your phone) that you can use to support integrating this new awareness practice into your life?

SHADOWS ARE HERE TOO

As you begin to cultivate greater self-awareness, don't be surprised if you bump into some shadow parts. You are bringing what is unconscious into your full consciousness, choosing to observe with clear inner vision the feedback within. Keep in mind that this may be followed by an uncomfortable period of hyperawareness. For instance, you might choose to bring awareness to the feedback that you're receiving around an addictive pattern you have (e.g., looking at your phone, compulsively eating candy, smoking pot, binge-watching). And then, suddenly, you'll see this same pattern everywhere in your life. It can be hard to stay present and observe without the self-judgmental parts getting activated. If that happens, circle back to the practices in Key #2.

If this feels familiar now, consider naming this pattern, describing it without justifying, apologizing, or getting stuck in a shame spiral. You might ask yourself the question: what is getting in the way of gentle, loving self-investigation right now?

TAKEAWAYS

✦ In your own words, describe what Key #3 means to you.

✦ What are three things you are taking away from this exploration with Key #3?

✦ What intentions do you have for the coming days, including any holding/support you may want to seek out?

BRINGING IT ALL TOGETHER

These first three keys interweave so much. Please, hold yourself with a kind, gentle heart as you open to all that your expanding awareness is bringing into your consciousness. There will be shadow parts that need tending. You will need courage and inner strength to stay with the discomfort that will inevitably arise, particularly when you are seeing things you'd rather not see. You may feel compelled to move on instead of lingering, or to try to "fix" what feels uncomfortable. If you can spend more of your time simply observing the patterns, the easier it will be to strategically address them in sustainable, life-giving ways.

And remember, you can only embark on your self-awareness exploration from where you are, not where you'd like to be. You can't be aware of everything at once. This is an ongoing lifelong practice.

This key is about shifting from searching outside for the answers to looking for and discovering them within. Once you have cultivated this kind of trust in yourself, you can then begin to seek out the support you need. You can begin to filter the outside input through your own self-knowing. Sustained habit changes start here through cultivating this depth of intimacy and self-awareness.

"You cannot control what happens to you, but you can control your attitude toward what happens to you, and in that, you will be mastering change rather than allowing it to master you."

—BRIAN TRACY

CULTIVATING RESILIENCE

The road to health and healing is rarely a straight shot or a smooth ride. The first three keys have paved the way, so to speak, by inviting you into an inner exploration, a way of getting to know yourself by honoring your life; by greeting your shadows and bringing them to light without shame; and by giving you the opportunity to consciously explore and open up to the internal feedback your body is sharing with you. At this point, you may be wondering, *And now what?*

This key, *Cultivating Resilience,* is designed to teach you how to take the internal feedback you receive and create real change in your habits, behaviors, and experiences.

There is no such thing as a stress-free or predictable life. Resilience is what allows you to pivot and adapt when something threatens to derail you—an accident, the death of someone you love, a troubling diagnosis, the loss of your job. Anything can happen at any time. You have no control over that. What you do have control over is how you respond. *Cultivating Resilience* guides you through an inner orientation, a realignment and re-direction of your state of being (physical, mental, emotional, and spiritual). This will empower you to consciously steer your-self toward your most alive self, regardless of what life throws your way.

EMBRACING CHANGE & UNPREDICTABILITY

In their book *Resilience Thinking,* Brian Walker and David Salt write, "At the heart of resilience thinking is a very simple no-tion—things change—and to ignore or resist this change is to increase our vulnerability and forego emerging opportunities. In so doing, we limit our options."[7]

Consider how you react when something has changed and caught you off guard. How does your body respond? What emo-tions rise to the top?

THE ROLE STRESS PLAYS

I can safely say that every single person I've ever worked with has named stress as a major contributing factor to the *dis*-ease they experience in their lives. So it makes sense to bring stress front and center for a moment. As we all know, stress is part of the human condition. Nothing we do will change that—nor should it. We can, however, learn how to meet our stress, diffuse it, and cultivate ways to bring our nervous system back into balance. Through such modalities as biofeedback, conscious breathwork and mindfulness practices—all ways to build inner resilience—we can shift our system out of a chronic sympathetic (fight-or-flight) state and into a predominately parasympathetic (rest-and-relax) state.

What stresses you out?

Let's try a little experiment. Let's see if it's possible to move from a stress state to a more relaxed state using your self-awareness muscles first—to receive feedback about how your body is responding—and then engage in practices designed to increase your resilience.

Begin by closing your eyes or softening your gaze. Let your mind wander until it lands on something that really stresses you out. It could be connected to your physical health, a relationship, your family, work life, the state of the world—really anything. Set the timer for three minutes and write down the story. As you are writing, can you feel the story in your body? Really feel all the feels connected to that experience. Name what you're feeling right now. How is your body receiving this information? Notice your pulse rate, your heartbeat, the temperature of your hands and feet, the rhythm, quality, and texture of your breathing. What is the state of your mind and emotions?

Now, pause. Try this breath practice and notice what happens.

Slowing your breath rate

When you're stressed, slowing your breathing can help calm your nervous system. Begin counting to five or six on your in-breath and five or six on your out-breath. Allow each in-breath to expand your abdomen and diaphragm and each out-breath to release them. Breathe like that for a couple of minutes, provided your breath feels smooth and easy (if it doesn't that's okay, just let the practice go for now).

Now, check back in with the state of your body—your pulse, your breath, the temperature of your hands and feet—and the state of your mind and emotions. What are you noticing now? What, if anything, feels different from before you did the breathing practices?

Take some time to reflect on all that you noticed before, during, and after this exercise.

ADDRESSING THE FEEDBACK

Reflect now on some of the takeaways for you from Key #3. Check in with your body. From the feedback it's giving you, what is feeling most relevant or urgent for you to attend to or take action around?

What skills, capacities, or knowledge might be most useful to engage with as you begin to address the inner feedback you have been gathering? What supports might you want to bring on board?

Is there a teacher whom you are curious to study with?

Is there a health practitioner who might have some tips or ideas of things you could do?

SKILL BUILDING & SELF-EDUCATION

With all of that in mind, here are some examples (just a taste!) of skills and knowledge you can actively learn. See if any items on the following list spark curiosity or inspire an initial direction for an exploration for yourself. Jot down notes of what comes to you.

Remember: Use your discernment about what *you* are drawn to. This list is not a homework assignment! There will be no quiz. These are simply suggestions on what you might consider exploring. Let your internal feedback guide your choices. *You* are your own best health guide.

Your anatomy and physiology

Consider taking a basic anatomy and physiology class to learn about how your miraculous body works! Or simply buy an anatomy and physiology coloring book and have some fun!

Structural integrity and flexibility

Help your nervous system and musculoskeletal system work more optimally by receiving bodywork, working with a personal trainer, or trying out some different mobility or movement classes (e.g., yoga, pilates, dance).

Digestion, nutrition, and eating

Learn about whole foods nutrition and how your digestive system works. Explore mindful eating. Take a cooking class. And, as Michael Pollan says, "Don't eat anything your great grandmother wouldn't recognize as food."[8] If you are particularly concerned about how specific foods might be affecting you, consider consulting with a trained holistic physician or nutritionist who can guide you through dietary changes.

Breathing

Your breath is the doorway through which you can shift your nervous system from a stressed fight-or-flight state to a more balanced rest-and-relax state. This form of self-regulation can impact your health and self-care on every level— your digestion, sleep, muscle tension, moods, and chronic illnesses. Consider exploring mindful breathing practices using an app, breath retraining with biofeedback (often uses a device and may be facilitated by a practitioner), or through studying with a yoga teacher.

Thoughts and emotions

When you consciously cultivate the capacity to shift your mental and emotional states, you can learn to shift the physiology of your body immediately. Explore different meditation, mindfulness, and yoga techniques. Take a dance class—or crank up the music at home—to move emotions through your body. Sing, chant, intone—using your voice to move sound and express your emotions is another excellent way to shift your internal state.

Sleep

Getting good quality and plentiful sleep is absolutely foundational to long-term health and well-being. Learn more about the restorative processes that happen in your sleep, how to optimize it, what sleep hygiene means, and how to create a sleep routine that works for you.

Elimination pathways

I encourage you to learn how to help your elimination pathways function more optimally each and every day—without focusing on detoxes and fasts. Your kidneys, intestines, liver, skin, lymphatic system, and lungs are all helping to let go of what you no longer need.

Hint: the most important thing you can do to support all of those systems is to drink lots of water! Additionally, help your body to sweat regularly, engage in physical movement, eat whole foods with lots of natural fiber, and receive massage and bodywork.

Relaxation and play

These days many of us need to learn (or relearn) how to have true downtime and engage in unstructured play. This is essential for your well-being. Choose activities just for the pure joy of doing them—no agenda allowed!—get silly, laugh out loud. Look to children if you need guidance, and experiment to discover what best helps you truly relax.

Exercise

Follow what lights you up, try new things, be social, get outside in nature, dance, let go of the "shoulds" and rejoice in moving and strengthening your body.

Sexuality

One of my mentor teachers said, "An orgasm a day keeps the doctor away!" Whether you are in a relationship or not, I highly encourage exploring and expanding your self-knowing in this way. Your sexual energy is your vital life-energy. Stoke that fire! And don't be shy; reach out for therapeutic support if you need it. This terrain can be ripe with shame and shadows for so many of us.

Attention

If you've noticed that your attention feels fragmented, and you find yourself multitasking, here are a few things to explore that may help you focus. Try out different forms of meditation, mindfulness practices, Qigong, or simply take yourself out for a mindful walk in nature. Experiment with technology-free times, as they can be significant healing influences these days in our over-stimulated attention.

CHECKING IN

Pause. Feel yourself in this moment. What's happening in your body? What emotions and thoughts are moving through?

Don't be surprised if you start spinning out a bit into some old patterns and ways of caring for yourself. This key can definitely bring that up. On the surface, it can read like a long list of "shoulds"—all the things you are "supposed" to do to take care of yourself. Take whatever time you need to embrace and attend to those parts that may have gotten stirred up (see Key #2).

Before you continue with your learning here, I suggest you bust out and throw a little dance party for yourself! Shake off the old ways, move the reactions through your body, connect with your joy and with some of those parts that have your back and are cheering you on!

TAKEAWAYS

✦ In your own words, describe what Key #4 means to you.

✦ What are three things you are taking away from this exploration with Key #4?

✦ What intentions do you have for the coming days, including any holding/support you may want to seek out.

BRINGING IT ALL TOGETHER

Cultivating Resilience is about the long haul. It is about responding to life's ever-changing reality—within you, your relationships, and the contexts you move through. Nothing is static. Whatever life throws your way, you can guide yourself from within that new reality toward a state that feels healthier, more alive, and more aligned with your well-being. Cultivating resilience allows you to adapt, dynamically steer, learn the skills and knowledge needed, and recalibrate to the new realities.

And cultivating resilience is an ongoing learning process. It is a practice of embracing that says, "Hey, I *want* to learn about these things! I want to expand my knowledge and skills! I want to seek out the supports and expertise to help me develop these capacities!" This is the embrace of the beginner's mind—curious, open, and eager to learn.

As you develop your own expertise, you discover an inherent ease and empowerment in caring for yourself. You come to see yourself as your own primary healer. You become masterful at guiding yourself, day in and day out, toward the most thriving, alive version of you that you can be.

"Run my dear,
From anything
That may not
   strengthen
Your precious
   budding wings."

—HAFIZ

ALIGNING WITH YOUR "YES!"

This key just might be my favorite. I know. I'm not supposed to have a favorite but I can't help myself. Aligning with my "yes!"? I'm all in. This key is all about cultivating a new inner guidance system for life that is rooted in the foundation you've cultivated so far with the other four keys. It's an invitation to consciously choose to invest your life-energy where you get returns and let go of anything that gets in the way of your natural blossoming.

I truly believe that *Aligning with Your "Yes!"* is the missing piece of the puzzle we need in relationship with healthcare. In the face of the statistics showing that burnout, fatigue, depression, anxiety, autoimmune conditions, and other chronic illness are on the rise, I have begun to believe that Key #5 is *the medicine we need most of all*. It's like the elephant in the room.

Can you envision living with the question, "Does this make me feel more alive?" as your orienting principle—your personal GPS? Consciously inviting in and moving toward your deepest yearnings and desires? *Aligning with Your Yes!* demands receptivity and agency. In other words, it asks that you be open to receiving inner guidance and then willing to take concrete steps in the direction you're being guided toward. Imagine feeling nourished on every level and able to trust that you are in the right place at the right time, doing what you are here on this planet to do. What would it take to give yourself full permission to thrive? What would it take to align with *your* "yes!"?

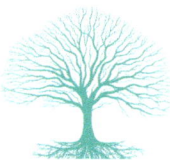

Check Your GPS

Your "yes" will change. Why? Because you are constantly learning, evolving, and growing. What feels aligned one day may no longer support you a week later. That's okay. Simply recalibrate from where and who you are at the moment—and let your inner GPS guide you.

INVESTING YOUR ENERGY

When you invest your life-energy where it feels aligned, you reap good returns—a deeper sense of vitality. And conversely, when you invest it where it doesn't align, you bear the cost of that—physically, emotionally, psychologically, and spiritually. Your investment might be completely unconscious (Key #2), but their impact is real. It is like a leaky boat, draining your life-energy away. Key #3 allows you to hone the awareness necessary to receive internal feedback, to notice how the choices you make affect you. When your choices are in alignment, the feedback you get is a feeling of being deeply nourished, alive, and present. When your choices are not aligned, you feel disconnected from your true nature. To paraphrase Abraham Maslow, if your essential core is denied or suppressed, you get sick. It may not happen right away, and it may not always be obvious, but it's often inevitable.[9]

Let's explore the ways in which you're investing your energy and how it's working (or not working) for you. I know it might feel like a lot, so take it slow, one question at a time, meeting each one with curiosity and grace.

✦ What brings you alive? When do you feel the most awake?

✦ In what ways are those things integrated into your daily life?

✦ What are ways you can prioritize aligning with your yeses more? What would support ytou in giving yourself more permission to do so?

✦ Where have you invested your energy that does not feel nourishing to you, that might even feel like a hole in your lifeboat?

✦ What are some of the ways you close yourself off from receiving what is nourishing and deeply aligned that might be currently available to you?

✦ There's a saying attributed to an ancient Chinese proverb: "Tension is who you think you should be. Relaxation is who you are." What does that mean to you?

DON'T POSTPONE YOUR "YES"

In her book *The Top Five Regrets of the Dying*, Bronnie Ware writes that the number one regret she heard as a palliative care worker was, *I wish I'd had the courage to live a life true to myself, not the life others expected of me.*[10] She goes on to say that "it's a pity that being who you are truly requires so much courage. But it does."[11] More than one hundred years earlier, Robert Louis Stevenson made a case for doing it anyway, when he wrote, "To know what you prefer, instead of humbly saying Amen to what the world tells you you ought to prefer, is to have kept your soul alive."[12]

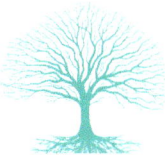

A Gentle Reminder
Aligning with Your "Yes!" *is not some kind of idealized reality. It's about being in direct, authentic relationship with the whole of who you are. Nothing is denied. It's not about getting rid of your pain, illness, struggle, or challenging emotions, or pretending they don't exist. It's about making space for them as you work to align your truth and your Yes! It's your truth and you own it.*

All of this is to say, give yourself full permission right now, without delay, to truly honor your own truth, your own intuition, your own calling—in other words, your "yes!"—regardless of what anyone else might think. Keep your soul alive.

The following questions can sometimes be hard to answer. Your mind may race to find the "right" thing to say, yet the real answer comes when you allow your mind to get out of the way and feel the answer fully in body and soul. You may find it helps to close your eyes and connect with your felt experience: What surfaces? Do you feel scared, vulnerable, excited? Honor each feeling, relax and trust in what emerges as you write using stream-of-consciousness.

✦ What matters most to you in your life? What do you yearn for on a soul level? Name it, even if it feels like it's too much to ask for or too good to be true.

✦ Close your eyes for a moment and feel what it feels like to unequivocally say yes to your deepest, most vulnerable desire (that maybe you have never uttered out loud to another person). What arises for you? Where do those feelings live in your body, your mind, and your heart?

✦ When do you feel that sense of deep alignment, like you are doing/being exactly what you're made for?

CHECKING IN

Close your eyes now and notice the emotions and thoughts that are swirling inside you. How and where do you experience those feelings in your body? Breathe into those sensations, letting yourself come into a deeper relationship with what is being stirred within.

And a reminder: As you touch into this territory, a lot of shadowy parts can get activated, both golden shadows and dark shadows. Are resistance and self-sabotaging thoughts showing up?

Circle back to Key #2 as you need to, and don't hesitate to reach out for the kind of support you may need.

PRUNING YOUR LIFE

I know this key is called *Aligning with Your "Yes!"* yet owning your authentic "no!" is at the heart of it all. One of my favorite metaphors for skillfully honoring your inner "no!" is to prune your life—much like you'd prune a fruit tree—delicately and mindfully. Not too much, not too little. The trick is to get rid of anything that is sucking the life out of the tree (such as branches that go straight up from the top of the tree and never flower or bear fruit); anything that is blocking the light (like extra branches growing on top of each other). When a tree is skillfully pruned, the whole tree flourishes, making way for organic blossoming and blooming to happen.

The same is true for you! When you prune the unnecessaries from your life—the things that no longer serve you—you make space for what aligns for you. The yeses. Consider the following categories as you begin your pruning process. I've offered a few examples for each one to help you seed your inquiry for yourself.

Physical belongings

If your material possessions no longer represent who you are now or are incompatible with the person you are becoming, it can feel like they are physically weighing you down. Take a look around your space and identify what no longer belongs. It could be anything—furniture, books, clothing, stuff you no longer use or like or have outgrown. Gather them up and give them away. You may be surprised at how much lighter you feel, and how little you miss any of it once it is gone.

Reflect: What physical belongings is it time to say goodbye to?

Household clutter

Having too much stuff cluttering your life—at home, at work, or in your car—can not only weigh you down, it can, according to a study done at UCLA, adversely affect your health and well-being. The solution isn't about merely thinning out your belongings; it's about facing your shadows, in the physical realm. You want to free yourself from what's literally getting in your way and blocking your light. You do this by creating order out of the chaos by organizing in such a way that each of your belongings has a home—a location that makes sense to you, and by recycling and donating what you can and throwing out the rest.

Reflect: Where in your home is there household clutter that needs tending to?

Volunteer commitments

There are so many ways to serve and offer your gifts in life. If you have said yes to something that's really a no, whether out of an obligation or a desire not to disappoint someone, let it go now! Free up your life-energy so that it is available for your unique callings.

Reflect: What volunteer commitments do you need to step away from or renegotiate?

Work

A tremendous amount of life-energy is invested in your work, regardless of what that looks like: full time or part time; stay-at-home parenting; or job hunting. Take a look at your work reality. Is it time to renegotiate the terms, such as work hours, schedule, or personal time off? Or is it time to step away, so you can create or find something that feels more fully aligned with your "yes!"?

Reflect: What in your work life needs pruning?

Relationships

Our relationships can be a source of so much nourishment and aliveness, or, if they are not aligned, a source of much dis-ease. This topic is too big and nuanced to get into here. So if you are leaning into more significant relationship pruning, please reach out for skillful support, whether that's from a professional or a loved one. A lot of shadowy parts are woven into this terrain, which makes discerning what is a true "no" confusing at times. Pruning relationships can sometimes be about shifting how you relate and how much, and learning and practicing healthy boundaries. Other times it is about letting go and saying goodbye.

Reflect: Are there any relationships in your life that are in need of pruning?

Home

Your home needs to be a haven for you, a place where you can feel safe, relaxed, renewed, and deeply nourished. What that looks and feels like is different for everyone. Take a look at your physical dwelling, its size and style, as well as its location, environment, and overall energy. Perhaps you long to be in nature, or in the heart of the city, instead of where you are, so a move is in order.

Reflect: What feels out of alignment for you in relation to where you live?

Beliefs

Although we touched into this in Key #2 when we brought unconscious beliefs, perspectives, and old patterns out of the shadows and into the light, it's time to revisit and acknowledge the importance of pruning anything that limits or prevents you from being in authentic, loving relationship with yourself. This includes any stories you have about yourself, your capacities, and who you could be. This step is imperative; you will not be able to move into alignment with your authentic self—or know what that feels like—without it.

Reflect: What are some beliefs that you're ready to prune?

Clearing internal space

This is a more subtle category of pruning, yet a vital step in aligning with your true nature. Because this level of pruning requires another deep dive into your shadows (Key #2), please take care of yourself and seek professional support when you need to. Clearing your internal space means acknowledging and releasing any unresolved tensions and emotions from your past that continue to take up space physically, mentally, emotionally, and spiritually long past their expire date. These are often attached to past traumatic experiences; they can zap your life-energy and cause chronic, debilitating health challenges. A few ways you can prune and clear your internal space on an ongoing basis include dancing, journaling, vocalization, somatic therapies, sexual release, and emotional release (give yourself full permission to cry when you need to).

Reflect: What are you holding onto from your past that you can begin to let go of?

When you have the courage to own your "no!" and let go of what no longer belongs or serves you, you get to live in receptivity, to see what is aligned for you now. So as you engage in pruning your life, circle back to these questions:

+ What or who is showing up in your life now that you have the space, and are ready and open to welcome them?

+ What did you have to prune from your life in order for your "yes!" to come to light?

Living in receptivity allows you to move through life centered in gratitude. From a grateful heart you can tune into, acknowledge, and connect more fully with your "yes!" What are you grateful for today?

TAKEAWAYS

✦ In your own words, describe what Key #5 means to you.

✦ What are three things you are taking away from this exploration with Key #5?

✦ What intentions do you have for the coming days, including any holding/support you may want to seek out.

BRINGING IT ALL TOGETHER

This key is about consciously creating and authoring your life by editing out what doesn't belong and inviting in what does. You are unleashing your vitality, releasing the energy that is caught in the heaviness and entanglement of what no longer belongs. This ongoing process of freeing yourself requires listening deeply and having the courage to be open to receive and prune as necessary. What emerges from this process? You feel alive at a deep level. You feel clear. You feel awake to and in contact with life's fullness. You are thriving!

Most of us yearn for more spaciousness in our lives, more breathing room. When you have the courage to prune your life and align with your "yes!" your life will begin to feel more spacious. And when that happens, you may find you are able to face your challenges head-on with tenderness, curiosity, and, yes, even gratitude. You don't have to live in a way that denies or invalidates your truth, that gets in the way of what is aligned for you. Instead, you can sleep, play, be held by others and hold yourself, rest more, and love more. And that's a helluva "YES!"

"At the height
of laughter,
the universe
is flung into a
kaleidoscope of
new possibilities."

—JEAN HOUSTON

EXPERIMENTING WITH PLAYFUL CURIOSITY

When I tune into this key, I get a felt sense of a weight being lifted off my shoulders. This key invites you to stop taking your health and self-care journey so seriously, to close the rulebook you may not even know was open. In other words, it's time to lighten up and start playing; put aside the "have-tos" and "must-haves," and instead embrace the "what-would-happens" of playful experimentation.

One of the best things about choosing playful curiosity in your self-care journey (and life) is there are no failures. Just one main rule of the game: Try things out and see what happens. By orienting yourself toward experimentation you take on an attitude of curiosity and active learning—because you never know for sure what the outcome will be. As you relax into framing your choices and intentions as experiments, rather than habitual "shoulds," you get to be a conscious, curious explorer of yourself, heeding the internal feedback you receive.

Why is all this important? Because so many of us have become trapped in an "I must do this to be healthy" prison, which has squashed our creative energy. What I mean is this: In trying so hard to be healthy, we have adopted *un*-healthy ways of relating to and guiding ourselves. We need an orientation to self-care that acknowledges that we're all constantly emerging; that nothing is static or linear. An orientation that puts less emphasis on finding answers and more on exploring possibilities. This softer, more feminine orientation is what this key is all about. It encourages imaginative experimenting. By channeling the spirit of playful curiosity, you get to find out what works for you and, equally important, what does not.

Experimenting with Playful Curiosity allows you to dance with your own emergence, the unfolding of your unique life story. You get to be playful, curious, childlike, exploring and learning as you go. Your health journey becomes an adventurous game. Life becomes a playground. And the freedom you experience in all of this becomes a huge part of your healing.

THE EXPECTATION TRAP

By now, you may already have a list of expectations that you must meet that dictate how well you're doing on your healthcare journey. You know the ones: "I need to stick to _____ if I want to be healthier." or "if only I could _____ then I'd be healthy." Here are some fill-in-the-blanks I hear often from clients:

"I need to stick to my diet and stop eating sweets if I want to be healthier."

"If only I could make myself go to bed by ten o'clock, then I'd be healthy."

"I need to stick to running every day if I want to be healthier."

"If only I could get myself to the gym and lift weights, then I'd be healthy."

I'd like to take a moment to bust the two most common myths of expectation. But first I invite you to explore some of your own expectations. Start with "I need to stick to [BLANK] if I want to be healthier." Set the timer for 1 minute and write down all the "need tos" you can think of. No censoring allowed!

Then move on to the statement, "If only I could [BLANK] then I'd be healthy." Set the timer for 1 minute and write down all the "If onlys" you can think of. No censoring allowed!

MYTH #1: THE "I NEED TOS"

The Myth of "I Need Tos." We unconsciously believe that in order to sustain the changes we seek we must not veer from "the Plan." Once we've determined what we believe *ought* to make us healthy, the Plan is now carved in stone. The corollary to "I need to stick to this diet or exercise routine if I want to be healthier" becomes "If I don't stick to this exact diet or exercise routine, I will never be healthy."

Caveat: This isn't to suggest there's no need for discipline; there is and we'll explore that in the next key. Or that there aren't exceptions, such as allergies that may cause us to go into anaphylactic shock, or health conditions that require certain protocols. There are, and we must take those seriously.

This is what I have found to be true. Having a plan that stays the same over time is not only unsustainable, it's the opposite of health. Firstly, it assumes that the routines and actions we set in place will always be what we need. Secondly, it doesn't take into account that we're forever evolving, growing, shedding the old and making room for the new, which is a natural part of life and imperative for a thriving vitality. And thirdly, it closes off our ability to flex our self-awareness muscles (Key #3) and align with our true "yes!"(Key #5).

We all have fundamental needs, yet there are myriad ways to nourish them. We each get to explore for ourselves how to do that over time (more on this later). We need an orientation to health that can flex and evolve along with us.

MYTH #2: THE "IF ONLYS"

The Myth of the "If Onlys." We believe if we just tweak the Plan by changing a particular behavior or cultivating a new habit, we'll feel healthy and be able to sustain the changes we seek.

Again, this sets us up for a whole lot of "shoulds." It invites tunnel vision that is focused on the particular—that one thing we now believe our plan lacks or that we lack the discipline for (likely a whole long list of them). This keeps us in an orientation toward our self-care that is about managing our bodies and our to-do list of things we need to do to be healthy. It also sets us up to be continually disappointed in ourselves.

Here's the thing: Our health is our *entire* lived experience. The details get to shift around as our life shifts around. Yet there is a ground that supports it all when we come into an entirely new relationship to health that can hold all of who we are, our entire life experience. To sustain the changes we seek, there needs to be *flexibility and adaptability*.

Reflect on what these myths reveal for you in your life:

What feels familiar for you in the descriptions of the myths? Does one stand out more than the other? How so?

How has your focus on the "I need to stick tos" and "if onlys" limited your perspective on your health and self-care? How has it shaped and affected your self-awareness and curiosity?

YOUR INNER GPS & ACTIVE LEARNING

Life is not static. Our resilience is in our capacity to navigate with fluidity and grace through the ever-changing realities of our existence. This key opens us up to embracing this movement of our lives with a spirit of adventure, curiosity, and playfulness. At any given moment, we get to listen, observe, and choose our next step. We can steer while in motion. We can try things out and experiment, while staying unattached to the outcomes; we get to learn as we go. Then we can decide on the next step, the next experiment. It sounds so lovely, so joyous. And yet . . . before we can fully commit to such playful experimentation, we need to acknowledge how hard it is to let go of the need to control the outcome and to begin to trust our internal GPS.

Consider the following questions:

+ What would it feel like to let go of trying to control the outcome, and allow your inner GPS to lead you? Describe the emotions that arise for you.

◆ What would support you in cultivating greater trust in your ability to steer yourself and learn as you go?

◆ In order to open more fully into the spirit of playful curiosity, what might you need to let go of, what might you need to grieve, acknowledge, or release first? And what are some of the ways you could do that?

✦ As you pivot toward playfulness and experimentation, what are some possibilities you'd like to explore for yourself?

✦ What do you think this key is beginning to reveal for you?

THE GAME OF LIFE

Let's take a moment here and acknowledge that no matter how hard we try, we're never going to figure everything out. I think it's fair to admit that none of us has any idea what this game called Life is all about. We're living in this big fucking miracle, fumbling around pretending that we have a clue, but we really don't. We're all kind of making it up as we go along. At least that's how it feels to me. And you know what? What that evokes in me is a sense of freedom.

Try this on with me here. Imagine you are living in the unknown, moving through life as an explorer—curious and open, with a spirit of adventure and playfulness. This is your journey right now. There's no rulebook, no Plan. You get to make it up as you go. Life is your playground.

What would being an explorer in your life mean right now? What does it evoke in you?

What would it be like for you to connect with a playful energy? How easy would it be for you to prioritize unstructured play in your life? What might be getting in your way?

Now pause (close your eyes if you like) and try connecting with your inner child; picture yourself as innocent and care-free, utterly consumed by this present moment. Feel how that feels. And then answer the following questions—staying in the mindset of your inner child:

What do you want to play around with in your life (or maybe simply in this moment)?

What do you want to try out just to see what happens, how it makes you feel, and how it impacts your sense of well-being?

CHECKING IN

Take a moment to pause, close your eyes, and let all of what you've been engaging with here sink in. Go outside if you can, take your shoes off, touch the earth, and feel your body and all the subtle signals letting you know you are alive. Notice what emotions are arising for you in this moment, and then let yourself open to the spirit of playful curiosity and see what bubbles up from within.

DESIGN YOUR FIRST EXPERIMENT

And now you get to design your first self-care experiment, by taking what you've explored on paper and putting it into practice.

Come to this experiment with playful curiosity, letting go of any expectation about the outcome or what "success" needs to look like.

To get you started, here are some examples of experiments others have done.

+ Turning off technologies at 8:00 every night—no phone, TV, or computer.

+ Decluttering-the-home sessions twice a week for 15 minutes, and starting it off with a dance party!

+ Doing five sun salutations each morning before getting dressed.

+ Eliminating refined sugar from the diet.

Some additional criteria to guide your creative process.

1. The experiment feels fun, nourishing, and unique to you.

2. It is something you haven't tried before.

3. Bonus points if you are able to meet multiple needs and nourishing things in one experiment. A weekly walk in nature with a friend, for example, means you've met your need for movement and gotten some social nourishment as well as nature nourishment.

Ready to play? Close your eyes now and listen for what feels like a priority for you at this time. What is one simple thing you could experiment with? If you are having difficulty tuning into this, flip back through your writing in the last couple of keys and see if any ideas are seeded that way.

Describe your first experiment here, then share it with your vitality buddy:

At the end of the two weeks, assess your experiment.

+ What felt good about it?

+ What didn't?

+ What was the hardest part about it?

+ What was the most surprising part?

+ What worked for you?

+ What if anything would you change in the experimental design?

Decide if you want to keep the experiment as is for another two weeks, tweak it, or scrap it completely and create your next two-week experiment.

CELEBRATING EACH STEP

Experimenting with Playful Curiosity allows you to notice and acknowledge the little steps that continue to open you into greater freedom, ease, and thriving; that keep you in dynamic movement and in alignment with your "yes!" Remember, this is about the long haul.

So in the spirit of that "yes!", take a moment now (and in an ongoing way) to celebrate those steps, no matter how small.

Make a list here of all that you have to celebrate right now:

Choose how to celebrate. You might share it with your vitality buddy? Throw yourself a little dance party? Go lie down on the grass and close your eyes? Or find another way unique to you to celebrate. Each time you do this, you anchor in this way of moving through your life, rooted in the 9 Keys to Deep Vitality.

TAKEAWAYS

✦ In your own words, describe what Key #6 means to you.

✦ What are three things you are taking away from this exploration with Key #6?

✦ What intentions do you have for the coming days, including any holding/support you may want to seek out?

BRINGING IT ALL TOGETHER

This orientation of *Experimenting with Playful Curiosity* acknowledges and supports that you are always in movement, dynamically steering into the unknown. You try one thing, and if it doesn't work, you try something else. You take in the data—recommendations, theories, and knowledge of others—and experiment with them. Try them on for size, see how they make *you* feel, and decide whether they fit into *your* unique flow and dance in life.

This key is where all of the other keys start translating into concrete actions in your life. Are you seeing how they all are building, one upon the next? In order to create your experiments, it is vital that you ground into an authentic relationship with where you are at this moment in time, to connect with your current realities, just as they are—not in some idealized idea of what you think your life is supposed to be, or what you have been projecting out there to other people, but actually landing fully in your truth. We'll be continuing to cultivate this grounding in the next key, *Key #7—Discovering Easeful Discipline.*

"There is
no freedom
without discipline,
no vision
without form."

—DAVID ALLEN

DISCOVERING EASEFUL DISCIPLINE

Sometimes when folks hear the word *discipline*, they think, *oh no, there goes all that playful curiosity and the fun, creative experimentation! Now we have to be more serious, more focused.* But easeful discipline actually goes hand-in-hand with the creative play we did in Key #6. They are intimate friends. Think of it this way: Playful experimentation creates the path toward this kind of discipline which, in turn, provides the necessary grounding and structure for creative play. As already mentioned, each key builds upon the other.

In order to sustain the changes you seek, you do need to practice discipline. *Easeful* discipline, the kind that comes with a fierce dedication to honor your unique life—fierce yet friendly and full of compassion. It's the kind of discipline that requires you getting real with yourself, doing what it takes to support your own thriving.

You need to be honest about all the obstacles, behavior patterns, contexts, people, and situations that trip you up and keep you from putting into action what would support your thriving. And then, like someone who truly has your back, you do what it takes to address each and every one—with intelligence, strategy, deep compassion, love, and, of course, playful experimentation!

UNPACKING THE D-WORD

Take a moment to consider what your relationship with discipline has been up until now—much like you did in Key #1 with the word "responsibility." Here are a few questions to start with:

+ When you read or hear the word "discipline," what is your immediate reaction? What feelings or thoughts surface?

+ Does the word evoke the inner Strict Parent part of you? Or perhaps the Rebellious Teenager inside? Or both? Is there another voice that feels familiar that shows up?

✦ What do those inner parts tend to say?

A D-word reframe

As you can see, so much of how we perceive discipline can get in our way of caring for ourselves in a conscious, nourishing way. How do we hold steady in our playfulness and still practice discipline? There's a quote by author Charles Eisenstein that, for me, really captures the essence of easeful discipline and what it's inviting us into. He says, "True discipline is really just 'self-remembering' . . . no forcing or fighting necessary."[13] Self-remembering. It's not about battling yourself into submission; it's about realigning with your commitments, with gentle yet fierce determination.

CHECKING IN

Pause for a moment and let yourself notice and feel into what may have come up for you in the inquiry around discipline. As you need, breathe into it, move with it, or sit with it. Take whatever time you need to embrace and tend to those parts that might be feeling the pain and grief for what your journey with discipline has been up until now.

Before we go any further, I just want to acknowledge that many of us have been battling ourselves into submission for years in our attempts to "be more disciplined." And as a result, shame can arise bigtime, particularly in relation to our self-care. We tell ourselves that we're not disciplined enough, or that we are weak and lack willpower. We tell ourselves that there is something wrong with us because we haven't been able to successfully enact and maintain the habit changes we want to make in our lives, the new realities we want to be living in.

It's not your fault! And it isn't an accurate reflection of who you are! You were never taught to engage with discipline in such a way that you could turn toward yourself with kindness and honoring. You haven't known how to do that. That is what you are learning here.

OLD HABITS DIE HARD

Why do we need discipline in the first place? Because it's not always easy to change long-standing habits and ways of being, even when we're fully committed. It takes time. And not only that, but the transitional period—out with the old, in with the new— can be really uncomfortable. It can take time to receive the clear internal feedback telling you that what you are doing is leading to more vitality. Discipline keeps us on track, steadily guiding us through the discomfort of change into a rebirth.

For instance, you might create an experiment to start jogging every day, after not doing it for months (or years!). At the beginning it doesn't feel good at all! It's hard to breathe, your muscles ache, and you're exhausted afterwards. These symptoms can make it really difficult to motivate yourself to continue. Or say you give up something—a particular food, substance, or person—you may experience a series of detox symptoms. You might feel sick, heartbroken, or confused. The transitional time might be longer than you want it or expect it to be, which is why you need discipline. It will keep you steady and engaged in the process.

The discomfort of change

Reflect back on a significant rebirthing or transition that took place in the past. It could even be a decision to change a particular habit. Name it in your mind and then take several minutes to engage with the following questions:

✦ What were some of the symptoms you experienced during that time? What parts of you were impacted—in your body, psyche, or spirit?

✦ How did the symptoms affect your day-to-day life? How did they affect your ability to stay with the change?

Now think about an intention for change you are currently leaning into. You can choose the focus of the experiment you created in the last key, or you might reflect on another one of the commitments that has shown up in your journaling earlier in this book. Sit for a moment and see if you can anticipate some of what you might experience in the early phases of the transformation you are seeking.

✦ What are the symptoms you're anticipating—physically, mentally, emotionally, and spiritually—when you are in that uncomfortable transitional time?

✦ What inner voices do you predict will be activated?

✦ When you bring those parts into your consciousness, what feelings or physical sensations surface?

PUTTING EASEFUL DISCIPLINE INTO PRACTICE

Easeful discipline is about self-remembering, realigning with and reaffirming your commitments. And it's about being *smart*. You will be rooting yourself in the orientations you have been cultivating in the other keys, so there is a sense of truly having your own back and loving yourself through the process.

I find that the best way to understand a new process is to actually do it! Just like in Key #6, you get to design an experiment. In order to find your way to successful, easeful discipline, you'll need to do the following:

1. Clarify your commitment

2. Create intelligent strategies

3. Implement structures of support

CLARIFYING YOUR COMMITMENTS

To be disciplined about something requires commitment; commitment requires that you get clear on what that something is. In previous keys, you have explored what some of your larger intentions are for your self-care journey (and your life!). You might revisit those keys now and see which of your priorities stands out to you or feels particularly relevant in this moment.

Once you home in on your larger intention, you will need to break it down into specific and doable steps or actions, like you did with the experiment in the last key. For instance, if you know that a priority for you is to feel energetic in your daily life, you might make some commitments around your sleep patterns, rest, play, or work schedule.

Or if you know that you come alive when out in the wilderness, you might set some intentions around taking more vacation time, scheduling a weekly hike, letting go of other commitments, or shifting your relationship to work.

Come up with a few commitments now that feel alive for you and list them here.

CREATING INTELLIGENT STRATEGIES

Next, pick one of your commitments related to something in your health journey you've tried to enact but have struggled to sustain. Ask yourself if this commitment would make you come more alive. In other words, avoid a commitment that feels like an abstract "should." Pick one that feels authentic—something you've been wanting to do but just haven't managed to make happen.

Using stream of consciousness, compose a list of obstacles that you suspect get in the way of you creating this change. Don't edit this; nothing is too silly or seemingly irrelevant. Capture everything that comes up for you.

Now transcribe each of those obstacles in the left column of this chart, and a potential creative solution or strategy to address each one in the right column.

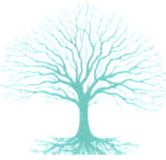

Caveat: *What we think of as obstacles are often competing commitments, real needs in disguise. See if you can hold each of them with curiosity and compassion, then find creative ways to meet these needs. There can be shadowy stuff here, too, that may need tending. You can think of this as creatively disentangling the competing commitments so that they are no longer in opposition to one another.*

Obstacles   *Creative Strategies*

IMPLEMENTING STRUCTURES OF SUPPORT

What do you need to put into place to support your success? Think of all the tools, programs, people, and rituals that might allow you to relax into your intentions and keep them front and center—with ease. These structures of support keep you in a container aligned with your commitments and values.

The following are some examples of such support structures. For each one, jot down any ideas that come to you that feel especially resonant with the commitment you are currently exploring.

Relational support

This is one of the most essential elements for succeeding in creating easeful discipline. Key #8 will explore this in depth; for now, consider a vitality buddy, professional support, a group, or a friend or loved one whom you trust to hold you in the depth of your journey and your commitments without judgment or shame.

Calendars

Get your commitments into your calendar. Consider them as planned dates with yourself, and treat them with the same level of integrity as you would an appointment with someone important (because, well, you are the most important person in your life!).

Rituals

Bring your creativity on board to design your own rituals that align with your commitments. For example, a morning walk on the trails to start the day with spiritual clarity and reflection or a candlelit soak in the bath each night to start your bedtime routine.

Programs

Engaging in a program that aligns with your commitment can be a way to bring an outside structure to your process, such as an online self-guided class, a local course, a book club, a retreat-based program, or a community sports league.

Reminders—love notes to yourself

The commitments you are making are as much a mindset shift as they are a habit change. Try putting up encouraging Post-it notes, images, or photos on your bathroom mirror, desk, bedside table, refrigerator, or front door that remind you in positive terms of your intentions. You can also have calendar reminders or screen-savers pop up on your phone or computer.

Inspiration

Find ways to stay connected to the deeper commitments you've made to yourself, to root back into what this is really about for you. Inspiring quotations, TED talks, audiobooks, or podcasts can help keep you inspired and connected to the bigger picture of this journey for you.

Shake it up!

If you find yourself getting stuck in seriousness and rigidity, shake it up! Dance parties, a playdate with your dog or cat, running around with a young child, giggle-fests to your favorite video clips, singing along to upbeat music, or wild, passionate sex (alone or with a lover) can all help you return to an open, relaxed, fluid place in how you are holding yourself in discipline.

WHAT'S YOUR NEW EXPERIMENT?

Now bring it all together and create a two-week experiment that draws on the previously mentioned steps: 1) clarify a clear commitment, 2) create strategies (flushing out all of the obstacles and getting real about how it will fit into your life), and 3) implement structures of support (choosing which ones to use and how you will use them).

Write down the details of your experimental design here:

TAKEAWAYS

✦ In your own words, describe what Key #7 means to you.

✦ What are three things you are taking away from this exploration with Key #7?

✦ What intentions do you have for the coming days, including any holding/support you may want to seek out?

BRINGING IT ALL TOGETHER

Active learning is at the core of discovering easeful discipline. It is not about getting it right. It is about learning as we go. It is about setting ourselves up as best we can to navigate through that uncomfortable transitional time of habit change until we get clear feedback affirming that what we are doing is life-giving for us (or not!). It's helpful to acknowledge that in those hard times of transition, we are gestating. That uncomfortable, in-between, liminal time is us being pushed through the birth canal. It is a rich creative space to be in, albeit disorienting—we can't yet see the new life waiting on the other side.

Easeful discipline is rooted in the foundation you have been cultivating since Key #1, a deep honoring of your unique life, a protective Mama Bear love that guides you to do what it takes to nourish and support your well-being, to have your own back. This foundation keeps you steady through the bumpy transitional times, keeps you patient through the learning process, and keeps you honest with yourself as you get real about the patterns at play and the real needs that are calling for your attention.

As you begin to put this key into practice, you may find that the time up front is an initial one-time investment: sorting out what your real commitments are, uncovering the real needs that are showing up as competing commitments, creating strategies to address those obstacles and needs, and creatively bringing structures of support on board. It will set you up to be able to truly live into your intentions more fully, to learn what works and what doesn't, and to disentangle from that boom-and-bust shame-ridden cycle. Applying a spirit of creativity, openness, curiosity, and playfulness to your commitments, strategies, and structures of support is what will bring the *ease* into the discipline.

"Life doesn't make any sense without interdependence. We need each other and the sooner we learn that the better for us all."

—JOAN ERIKSON

INVITING SUPPORT AND CONNECTION

Before my health crisis in my mid-twenties, I was fiercely independent. If someone were to even suggest that I reach out and share my fears and vulnerabilities with others, I'm pretty sure that wouldn't have resonated with me. I wasn't even aware that I needed support. Then life brought me to my knees and I learned otherwise. I had no choice but to ask for what I needed. As a result, this key—*Inviting Support and Connection*—became a HUGE part of my healing journey.

Inviting Support and Connection is all about coming out of isolation. It's about recognizing that you can't do your health journey alone. No ingredient is more powerful and essential to actualizing the full potential of your thriving than relational support. We are relational creatures—we need each other.

When you truly commit to stepping onto this path and embracing your authentic self (*Key #1—Honoring Your Unique Life*), leaning into others for support gets easier. Why? Because you feel such fierce self-love and loyalty, that you'll do whatever it takes to heal. You're willing to face and embrace the shadows that may have gotten in the way of you reaching out for support and connection before. You're willing to share the most vulnerable parts of yourself in service to that healing.

LOOKING WITH CLEAR EYES

When you think about the relationships in your life—with your friends and colleagues, with people you love and respect—it can feel so life-giving to connect and cultivate intimacy. And yet if you're like many of us, you'll find you're more willing to share the safe parts, the funny parts, the more universally accepted parts of your story and leave out the "cringe-worthy" vulnerable parts that reveal your humanness and shame. Of course, by keeping parts of our lives separate (as dominant culture encourages us to do), our shame can become compounded: *Something is wrong with me. No one else understands what this feels like* . . . and on and on it goes.

Take a moment to reflect on the connection and support you have available in your life right now. How does it show up (or not) in relation to your health and self-care journey? Write down your answers to the following questions without overthinking.

Are there friends you feel comfortable sharing only certain aspects of your life? Do you have friendships (or love relationships) in which you feel safe to share your vulnerable side, but not the more sensitive aspects of your self-care journey? Maybe you would like to share more but you're afraid of being judged. What holds you back from sharing more?

Is there anyone in your life now with whom you can share your deepest vulnerabilities and shame? Describe the qualities of your connection with that person that sets it apart from other relationships. What is it about that person that creates a sense of safety for you.

Based on how you describe the types of relationships you have, spend a few minutes writing the answers to the following questions: What do you receive from the connections you have? What do you contribute? What kinds of support would you like to receive from your relationships but currently aren't?

THRIVING THROUGH CONNECTION

Connecting with others gives us the support we need to heal and thrive. Here are several ways we can benefit from relational support.

Reflections

As we learned when working with Key #2, we can't possibly see everything about ourselves by ourselves. We need perspective and the feedback from others we trust so we can uncover old beliefs and paradigms we've been operating from without even realizing it. Others can help us bring the unconscious into the conscious, the shadow to the light.

Look back at Key #2 now, or some of the other journaling you have done around shadow work. What areas of your life or self-care journey do you believe would benefit from having this kind of support, support that will help to reveal what you haven't been able to see for yourself?

Skill and capacity building

Don't be afraid to seek advice from others in your community. Intentionally reaching out to teachers, guides, programs, and classes will strengthen your self-awareness and help you cultivate new skills and capacities.

Look back at your notes from Key #3 and Key #4. Consider what is relevant to you right now. What types of skill and capacity-building support would you like to seek out at this time?

Guidance

We can't know what we don't know. Luckily there are those we can reach out to who have walked these paths before, those who are familiar with territories we never even knew existed. These vital guides and mentors can orient us, let us know what to expect, warn us of roadblocks and pitfalls, and get us started on our own journey.

Are you in the midst of a transitional time? Do you have a sense of moving into the unknown, into territory you're unfamiliar with? Think of someone whom you look up to, someone who embodies the life experiences you haven't had yet (or that you are in the midst of). Maybe this is a mentor who is further along on their journey. How might they support you in your life now? What questions might you ask them? What is holding you back from asking for their guidance?

Accountability

There's nothing quite like being accountable to another person or group of people when you're experimenting with—and sometimes struggling to maintain—life changes. Having that kind of reliable support has been the magic ingredient for me; it's always made a huge difference in my life.

What are you attempting to change in your life that might benefit from greater accountability (the kind, loving variety)? You might look back at the experiment you created in Key #7 as a starting point.

Love

Never underestimate the power of love to get to the heart of what needs to be healed. Truly, nothing is more transformative than being held, than receiving the kindness and compassion of others. What seems unreachable is suddenly within grasp. Giving your full attention to someone else with loving care can also help heal you.

When you imagine inviting a loving embrace into your journey, what images, feelings, and realities are evoked for you? Are there any hesitations that linger?

Perspective

Being part of a larger unfolding can put things into perspective in a way that helps you remember that you're not alone, that you're part of something bigger than yourself, and that your health journey is not just about you. We'll be returning to this in *Key #9— Living Like You Matter.*

When, with whom, and in what context do you notice yourself popping out of a smaller "me" orientation and into feeling a deeper connection with others, with life as a whole? What helps you remember that your life and your well-being are not just about you?

CHECKING IN

Take a moment to pause. As you breathe into the present moment, what is arising for you? How does it feel when you welcome the support of others? To offer your support? Check in with your heart, your mind, and your body. Is anything wanting to move, unwind, release, or open in your body or your being?

WHO IS ON YOUR SUPPORT TEAM?

Embarking on anything new requires creating a *team* of support you feel comfortable with. Such a team often includes professional expertise as well as family members, partners, and peers. No one person can give you everything you need to thrive. I've seen time and again how powerful it is when we consciously create our support team, people who can stand behind us and with us in explicit ways. I've listed a number of categories for you to consider as you build your own team.

Peer support

Remember when I suggested having a vitality buddy join you in this journey, someone you know and trust, who is also prioritizing their own healing and transformation? This is where they come in! Peers can offer accountability, love, perspective, and even guidance when you're wavering or feeling overwhelmed. Look for a buddy who is going through something similar or is ready to make changes in their own life. You can even have several vitality buddies—one for every commitment you are leaning into and every experiment you are playing with! Use your creativity and the spirit of experimentation to find what works best for you.

Caveat: Always make sure it is mutual support, that you stay within the appropriate boundaries for peer support and seek out professional help to complement it as needed. You might consider meeting up a couple of times a week to exercise and check in; text each other your intentions each morning and a wrap-up of the day each night; create a weekly time to journal and share your reflections with one another (perhaps with *The Vitality Journal* or *The Vitality Map*).

✦ What do you need right now that a vitality buddy can support you in? How best can this person support you? How best can you reciprocate?

✦ Think of a person you might want to explore a conscious peer support relationship with. What are some of the qualities that make them a good choice?

✦ What are some ways you might support one another?

Partner/family

Your romantic partner and members of your family can often be amazing sources of support. There is the added benefit of living under the same roof or having your lives already woven together in some ways, making intentional collaboration and encouragement potentially easier to integrate. Tread lightly here, though, and with tenderness and clarity. Every relationship is different; you and your partner or family member may not always be in alignment. Sometimes the timing is off or life priorities are too different. Please don't assume anything, keep the appropriate boundaries and expectations in mind, and work together to discover what might serve you both.

+ Imagine inviting other dimensions of conscious mutual support into your romantic partnership or family relationships. What comes up for you? Any trepidation? Excitement? Inspiration? Anxiety? Creativity?

+ What aspects of your self-care journey do you think would benefit from this kind of mutuality? Take the lid off and let your imagination dream into the possibilities and see what arises.

◆ Which person in your family do you feel most aligned with right now? How would it feel to ask for their support?

◆ What are some potential challenges in bringing your partner or family into your process? What sorts of boundaries do you think you'd need to make this a fruitful connection?

Healthcare professionals

This is a huge category, one ripe with possibilities for all kinds of support. Different types of professional support will be relevant to you at different times, for different reasons, and with different frequencies. Remember that this is a *one-way relationship*; that means you are hiring them to be of support to you, without any of the other complexities of relationship or any need for you to reciprocate. It's up to you to be discerning, and to have your own back when choosing whom to work with. You are in charge of your health journey, and these health professionals work for you. If at any time you are not feeling heard or respected, let that person go and seek out another practitioner. Some examples of professionals you may want on your team:

+ conventional doctors and specialists

+ naturopathic physicians

+ acupuncturists

+ psychotherapists and coaches

+ chiropractors, bodyworkers, somatic therapists, personal trainers

+ nutritionists

When making your list, consider these questions:

+ What kinds of professional expertise and holding would be of support to you now?

◆ What qualities would you like to look for in the healthcare professionals you invite onto your team? Consider the following qualities: how they listen, see, and relate to you; how their energy affects you emotionally when you are with them; the quality of their presence; their capacity to be with complexity, vulnerability, shame, and other emotions.

◆ Are there any healthcare professionals currently on your team of support whom you don't resonate with, who do not embody the qualities you are seeking?

Medical advocates

Although you are your own best health guide, there may be times (maybe even now?) when you're not able to confidently weigh your choices and options. Perhaps you are in the midst of navigating a serious illness or are feeling confused by the healthcare system and your current team of doctors. A medical advocate can be your partner, a family member, friend, or a paid professional, who comes with you to your appointments, asks questions, takes notes, and helps you keep track of your journey when you're in the throes of anxiety, brain fog, and overwhelm. Who would feel like a trusted companion to support you in this way when/if you need it?

Community of practice

So many of us long for deep communion, for safe spaces where we can be our glorious and messy selves, lovingly explore our complexities, hear the stories of others going through similar experiences, and realize that we are not alone. Our stuck parts relax and our vulnerabilities shift when we're held in a safe, contained, intimate, and confidential healing group. In my experience there is nothing more powerful to catalyze healing than intentionally coming together like this. Healing begins when we emerge from our isolation; it continues by seeing and being seen, hearing and being heard, sharing our shame stories and vulnerabilities with others and listening to their stories in return. For intentional "communities of practice" to work, it's vital that you feel held in a *safe* healing space. You must *trust* the holding and facilitation, trust that you and the other participants come together around a set of agreements that are rooted in honor, respect, confidentiality, and an acknowledgment of the wholeness, autonomy, and capacity of each individual. Reflect on any experiences you have had in a group program focused on personal growth and healing—or in an intentional community of practice, even if it's not related explicitly to health or self-care.

+ How did the group experience serve you? What did it offer that a solo practice, learning experience, or one-on-one support could not?

+ What worked for you in the facilitation? What did you yearn for that perhaps wasn't met in how that group was held?

✦ What sort of community of practice might you feel drawn to now? What topics or themes would you want to explore with others? What do you feel like needs a deeper container of support and reflection with a community of peers?

Now that you have explored the various types of supports you might invite onto your team, let's bring it all together to create a clear plan:

✦ Describe specifically what type of support you need and what role each person would play on the team. Make a list of the roles you want to fill.

✦ Make another list of people you already know who might fit these roles. And then list the people you think may be able to offer recommendations or referrals.

✦ Who on these lists do you feel comfortable reaching out to right away?

TAKEAWAYS

✦ In your own words, describe what Key #8 means to you.

✦ What are three things you are taking away from this exploration with Key #8?

✦ What intentions do you have for the coming days, including any holding/support you may want to seek out.

BRINGING IT ALL TOGETHER

The foundation of *Inviting Support and Connection* is that you acknowledge the following: You are your own best health guide. Turning to others for support is not about handing over your authority or power, and it is not about needing to be fixed in any way. Instead, it is an act of strength, an honoring of your unique life, a recognition that in order to thrive you need to be held by others too. And you run that support—the guidance, knowledge, skills, and capacities you are learning— through the filter of your own self-knowing. You take in what serves and release the rest.

It is essential for this key that you cultivate your capacity *to trust in your own discernment*, to have the courage to create a team of support that aligns with *your* values. Your healing journey includes vulnerabilities, shadows, and shame. It's imperative that those on your team have the capacity to hold all of who you are—the darkness and the light—with sensitivity, gentleness, love, and compassion.

As Brené Brown cautions in *The Gifts of Imperfection*, "If we share our shame story with the wrong person, they can easily become one more piece of flying debris in an already dangerous storm."[14] However, in her book *Daring Greatly*, she also writes that "if we can share our story with someone who responds with empathy and understanding, shame can't survive."[15]

All of the other keys have helped increase your capacity to truly lean in, embrace, and rejoice in a circle of support. And as Key #8 weaves the rest of the keys together into a whole, you are reminded again and again that no one can journey alone. As relational creatures, we humans need each other. In consciously creating your team of support, may you feel a huge opening and shift in your capacity to care for yourself and may that guide you into greater resilience and well-being.

"Don't ask yourself what the world needs. Ask yourself what makes you come alive and then go do that. Because what the world needs is people who have come alive."

—HOWARD THURMAN

LIVING LIKE YOU MATTER

As we arrive at this final key, we've come to appreciate that we don't heal alone, that we need each other. And now we deepen further into the realization that our vitality and personal well-being is intimately connected to the health and well-being of our communities, the planet, and to all of life.

Here's the truth: Each of us has a role to play in creating a positive future for everyone. In order to step into that role, however, we must stay as strong, clear, and vital as we can. *Living Like You Matter*, the ninth and final key in your health and self-care journey, is an invitation and a call to action for you to consciously cultivate the foundation in yourself that you need to serve others.

We face stark realities as a human family. In this time of rapid change with so much challenge and complexity, it can feel like our individual, collective, and planetary health is teetering in the balance. True service is rooted in nourishing and stewarding your own body and being into your most alive, vital version of you, so that you can unleash your unique creative offering on the world. This is living like you matter.

THIS MOMENT IN HISTORY

There is so much need in our world now, so much disease individually, collectively, and globally. And the realities we are navigating as a human family are taking their toll on us all. Epidemics of burnout, exhaustion, depression, anxiety, and so many other manifestations of chronic stress-related illnesses are the norm these days. Add to that the isolation many of us are living in and the existential angst so many of us feel in the face of climate change, loss of species, human conflict, and more, and it is a wonder we are functioning at all!

✦ How are you doing with it all? How are the bigger realities we are living in impacting your sense of well-being?

✦ What does it catalyze or clarify in you?

✦ What does all of this have to do with living like *you* matter?

THE BODHISATTVA SYNDROME

It is natural and honorable to feel the impulse to do our part, to be of service in the face of so much need. And yet in our eagerness to help, we can find ourselves disconnected from our own needs, from tending to our own well-being. For many of us it can be so much easier to care for others than to care for ourselves, to show up in support for those around us than to ask for what we need ourselves. We end up ultimately sacrificing the things we most love in order to make a difference. Here's the thing though: Although you may be helping others, you are not living like *you* matter.

In Buddhism, a bodhisattva is someone who devotes their life to reducing the suffering of all sentient beings. I have playfully come to refer to the all-too-common pattern of prioritizing care for others at the expense of caring for ourselves as the Bodhisattva Syndrome. It is heartbreaking to see how entrenched these beliefs and behavior patterns can be, how reinforced they are culturally. In neglecting to include ourselves in our bodhisattva vow, in not caring for our own life as we do others, we have less to offer, less capacity to show up in support for others and our collective future. Everyone loses.

This people-pleasing, self-sacrificing orientation can easily undermine your vital well-being. Why? Because in your earnest desire to compassionately serve others, you have forgotten to care for yourself.

Does this ring true for you? Take a moment to think about how and when you prioritize the needs of others above your own—and with whom. And then explore the following questions and observe what arises:

✦ How does it feel to put your own needs aside for others? What is the impact on your well-being?

✦ How does that make you feel about yourself?

✦ Where do you feel the impact the most in your relationships?

✦ What do you see as the longer-term impacts if you continue with these patterns?

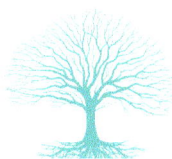

"The person you'll have the hardest time opening to and truly loving without reserve is yourself. Once you can do that, you can love the whole universe unconditionally."[16]
—Adyashanti

Living Like You Matter is all about healing the split between caring for yourself and serving the greater good. It's the way to be a bodhisattva in this life *without forsaking yourself.* This is imperative if you are to thrive.

✦ What might your life look like if you no longer sacrificed yourself in order to serve? Describe a scenario in which you could serve or care for someone without sacrificing your own needs and desires. How would that be different? How do you think it would change how you showed up?

✦ What would you need to change in order to serve others while also honoring your own health and well-being?

The thing is, when you step into compassionate service without losing yourself, you acknowledge and experience the interconnectedness of all beings—in real time. As Fritjof Capra said, "We have to regain our experience of connectedness with the entire web of life."[17]

CHECKING IN

Pause now and check in with yourself. You might close your eyes and feel all the ways you can sense that life is pulsing through you—in the beat of your heart, the rhythm of your breath, the warmth of your hands. Now tune in more subtly to what it feels like to be alive and in a body, to the exquisite awareness of life infusing every tiny cell within you, every thought, every feeling, and to the awareness that is able to hold it all.

Now expand that awareness outward. Tune into the other people around you as if you were following a thread of a web, beginning with those closest to you, expanding out to those far away, to those whom you have never met. Focus on the deep connection you feel with those in your human family and how life is infusing you all. Extend your awareness to the animal and plant life around you, then slowly widen it to include all life on the planet.

Come back now to your own body and the pulsations of life moving through you. Feel the ways that same life-energy moves through the entire web of life.

Take a moment now to write down what arose for you in that check-in meditation.

SERVING LIFE

Remember back to *Key #1—Honoring Your Unique Life*. When you really understand that key—not intellectually, but physically and spiritually—it translates not only to your relationship with self-care, but how you show up in the world. You are utterly unique, the only expression of life like you there is. There is no accident in you being here. When you show up as you—as vital, as alive, and as self-expressed as you can be (regardless of what you are navigating)—you are serving life. What matters is that you are the one blossoming and blooming in the world in ways that are aligned with your "yes!"

There are no hard and fast rules on how to be of service. Your only obligation, as Bill Plotkin writes, "is to reach as deeply as you can and offer your unique and authentic gifts as bravely and beautifully as you're able."[18] Remember, too, that being of service can happen in all spheres of your life, with the impacts felt close to home, or around the globe—your professional work, parenting and caregiving, a volunteer project, the way you interact with and acknowledge strangers in the grocery store, or how you lend a hand to neighbors in need. It's how you, with your talents and your unique gifts, make the world around you a better place.

Living Like You Matter invites you to choose life, choose to thrive, so that you may serve others in the way that only you can. Our world needs you! You matter. As you come to the end of this key, let the following questions guide you toward the fullest expression of yourself, one that allows you to bring forward your unique contribution to the world.

✦ Set a timer for 3 minutes. Write the words "Living like I matter" at the top of your page, then freewrite. Don't try to control your thoughts; don't edit. Simply write.

Living Like I Matter

✦ If you were to give yourself full permission to align with your "yes!" when it comes to your service in the world—to live from "I get to" rather than "I have to"—what might that look like?

✦ Who or what would you be impacting, touching, or supporting with your unique presence, your unique gifts?

✦ If you allowed yourself to really be seen, to really show up in the world with your full presence, what might that look like? What would that change in your life? What feelings are evoked in you in that imagining?

✦ How might you align your ways of serving others with your own self-care so that you come more fully alive in your creative offering? What would fill your well?

✦ What experiment could you create that would explore the interconnection between your own sense of vitality and the ways in which you show up to serve others?

✦ What's one action step that you could take today to step more fully into living like you matter?

TAKEAWAYS

✦ In your own words, describe what Key #9 means to you.

✦ What are three things you are taking away from this exploration with Key #9?

✦ What intentions do you have for the coming days, including any holding/support you may want to seek out.

BRINGING IT ALL TOGETHER

Please remember that *Living Like You Matter* isn't about putting pressure on yourself to single-handedly save the world (or whatever your version of that may be). It is about acknowledging you have gifts that no one else can offer the way that you can; that you are a unique expression of life; and that your personal unfolding is *life* unfolding.

It is up to you to listen and tune in to what lights you up, to how you want to invest your life-energy in ways that support your own thriving, and uniquely nourish you on an ongoing basis. This isn't about *fixing* yourself or living up to some ideal. When you care for yourself in these ways, the self-care extends beyond the *self.* The distinction between individual, collective, and planetary healing drops away. You are serving life, of which you are a vital part. When you support your own blossoming, blooming, and thriving, when you allow your unique life expression to shine in the world, regardless of who, what, or how it is showing up and touching others, this kind of self-care *is* living like you matter.

A LETTER
IN CLOSING

Let's pause to reflect on the journey you've been on, what you've done, what you are choosing, where you are now, and what it took to get here. You have arrived here at the end of this journal. Let it sink in. What are you feeling in this moment?

I want to acknowledge with you the courage and inner strength it takes to keep turning toward yourself in the ways you've been doing with *The Vitality Journal*: to come home to yourself; to be with your vulnerabilities; and to accept, love, hold, and tend to all the different parts (including the shadowy ones). And not just to choose once, but to choose again and again, to be awake and aware and in contact with it all.

While it feels important to acknowledge that you completed your work here, this is not really the end. It is just the beginning of a journey you can live into for the rest of your life. You have been consciously cultivating a new foundation, a new operating system, and a new way of holding and guiding yourself. This approach is now *yours* to utilize throughout your lifetime.

The wonderful thing about the nine keys is that they will grow along with you. They will translate and be relevant to you in changing life circumstances, shifting priorities, and stages of life—and as you continue to evolve, discover, and become.

When you are ready, come back to this journal here to keep exploring. If you want a deeper dive, read my book *The Vitality Map*—available in audiobook, ebook, or paperback versions (TheVitalityMap.com).

And . . . I'm here for you. Reach out and lean in for support and connection. I have virtual and retreat-based group offerings as well as one-on-one support for varying levels of engagement and need. Visit VitalMedicine.com to learn more.

I want to leave you with some sentiments that are close to my heart and my wishes for you, for myself, and for all of us:

+ May you continue to find your way home to yourself, to this unique expression of life that you are. And that you honor and love yourself, garden and tend to yourself as if you are the most precious being alive (which, to you, you are!).

+ May you continue to connect with your courage and strength within; to accept, embrace, and own all of who you are with empathy and compassion, while inviting those parts of you that have been in the shadows to join you at the table.

+ May you continue to tune in, listen for the feedback your life-energy is giving you in every moment, and choose to become more intimate with yourself—you will become more adept and skillful at guiding yourself toward your most resilient, thriving self.

+ May you say "yes!" to your "yes!" Open to the life that is here for you to live, to who you are here to be; prune away what no longer serves you; and clear the impediments to your natural blossoming and evolution.

+ May you let your inner wild one out to play—dance, move, and flow with life. Embrace caring for yourself in the spirit of curious wonder, and as a sweet, playful experimentation. Remember there is no such thing as failure. You learn and reorient as you go, trusting in the unfolding, listening for what wants to happen next . . . opening and allowing.

+ May you do what it takes to have your own back, to guide yourself through disorienting transitions by following clear commitments, savvy strategies, and putting in place all of the supports you need!

+ May you invite a circle of support around you, those who you feel safe with, who can hold your vulnerability, shame, and shadowy parts with the kindness, empathy, and love that they and you need and deserve.

+ And may you truly get, in the deepest realms of your being, that *you matter* and then take the lid off of your life and LIVE that way!

ENDNOTES

1 Joanna Macy, "Personal Guidelines for the Great Turning," accessed May 26, 2015, http://www.joannamacy.net/personal-guidelines.html.

2 A. Mille, *Martha: The Life and Work of Martha Graham* (Random House, 1991), 264.

3 Mary Oliver, "The Summer Day" from *New and Selected Poems* (Beacon Press, 1992).

4 Bernie S. Siegel, *Love, Medicine and Miracles: Lessons Learned about Self-Healing from a Surgeon's Experience with Exceptional Patients* (HarperCollins, 2011), Kindle Edition, 67–68.

5 Steven Pressfield, *The War of Art* (Black Irish Entertainment LLC, 2011), Kindle Edition, 12.

6 Marianne Williamson, *Everyday Grace* (Riverhead Books, 2002), 12–13.

7 Brian Walker and David Salt, *Resilience Thinking: Sustaining Ecosystems and People in a Changing World* (Island Press, 2006), 9.

8 Michael Pollan, *In Defense of Food: An Eater's Manifesto* (Penguin, 2008), 148.

9 Abraham Maslow, *Toward a Psychology of Being* (John Wiley & Sons, 1999), 6.

10 Bronnie Ware, *The Top Five Regrets of the Dying: A Life Transformed by the Dearly Departing* (Hay House, 2012), Kindle Edition, 214.

11 *Ibid.*, 213.

12 Robert Louis Stevenson, *The Novels and Tales of Robert Louis Stevenson: An inland voyage. Travels with a donkey*, Edinburgh (Charles Scribner's Sons, 1895), 17.

13 Charles Eisenstein, *The Yoga of Eating: Transcending Diets and Dogma to Nourish the Natural Self* (New Trends Publishing, 2003), 4–5.

14 Brené Brown, *The Gifts of Imperfection: Let Go of Who You Think You're Supposed to Be and Embrace Who You Are* (Hazelden Publishing, 2010), Kindle Edition, 10.

15 Brené Brown, *Daring Greatly: How the Courage to Be Vulnerable Transforms the Way We Live, Love, Parent, and Lead* (Penguin Publishing Group, 2012), Kindle Edition, 75.

16 Adyashanti, *Falling into Grace* (Sounds True, 2011), Kindle Edition, 229.

17 Fritof Capra, *The Web of Life* (First Anchor Books, 1996), 96.

17 Bill Plotkin, *Nature and the Human Soul* (New World Library, 2010), 376.

ABOUT THE AUTHOR

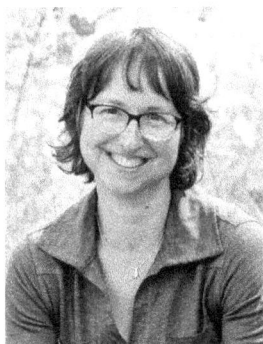

Dr. Deborah Zucker is a naturopathic physician, mental health counselor, health coach, and the award-winning author of *The Vitality Map: A Guide to Deep Health, Joyful Self-Care, and Resilient Well-Being.* She specializes in empowering individuals to cultivate embodied compassion and a deeper understanding of what truly ignites their vitality. With her guidance, clients consciously design their unique transformation—embracing freedom, confidence, and ease as they learn to follow their heart toward healing and renewal.

It was Dr. Deborah's own journey with chronic illness that evolved into a calling to support others in their healing. Over the years, her personal and professional experiences have engendered an intimate understanding and humility for the ways in which life can bring us to our knees. She deeply knows the courage and resilience it takes to emerge from life's intense transitions, to navigate one's own authentic path in life, and the profound need for skillful *and* loving support on that journey. This is her heartfelt passion and mission.

Dr. Deborah guides clients to discover a path to greater alignment with who they are here to be and what brings them uniquely alive. Through Vital Medicine, she offers transformative women's circles, one-on-one coaching and counseling, retreats, and her signature program, Vital U. Connect with Dr. Deborah online at VitalMedicine.com.